TOTAL HEALTH

D1475373

PETER BURWASH

TORCHLIGHT PUBLISHING INC.
BADGER, CA, USA
KOLKATA, WEST BENGAL, INDIA

Cover and book design by Kurma Rupa/Mani deep
Printed in India

Published simultaneously in The United States of America and
Canada by Torchlight Publishing Inc.

Library of Congress Cataloging-in-Publishing Data
Burwash, Peter
        Total Health : the next level : a simple guide for taking control
of your health and happiness now! / by Peter Burwash
                p.   cm.

        Includes bibliographical references.

        ISBN 1-887089-10-1
        1.Health.   2. Nutrition.   3. Vegetarianism.. I. Title.
    RA776.B9526   1997   97-16674

    613- -dc21

**Attention Colleges, Universities, Corporations, Associations and
Professional Organizations:** *Total Health* is available at special discounts
for bulk purchases for promotions, premiums, fund-raising or educational
use. Special books, booklets, or excerpts can be created to suit your
specific needs.

For more information contact the Publisher
Torchlight Publishing, Inc
PO Box 52
Badger CA 93603
Email: torchlight@spiralcomm.net
www.torchlight.com

Dedication

To my eldest daughter, Kimberly:

May this book help protect and preserve all your friends—those in the human world, those in the animal world, and those in the plant world—for we're all woven together in the same and splendid kingdom.

Acknowledgments

My sincere thanks to all those who shared their time and expertise in bringing this book to completion. A special thank you to Susie Hodges for typing the manuscript, Larry Kahn for its initial editing, and Dr. Michael Klaper for reviewing the medical references.

Praise for
Total Health: The Next Level

"Peter Burwash really hits the nail on the head: What we eat is the single largest influence on our bodies! Total Health *opens the curtain on food preparation and gives you a chance, perhaps for the first time in your life, to see clearly what gives you the edge and which foods poison your body, mind, and soul. This book is terrific and long overdue."*

Ingrid E. Newkirk
President, PETA
(People for the Ethical Treatment of Animals)

"Peter Burwash serves up another ace. Once again Peter demonstrates his ability to simplify the complex, while others complicate the simple. Just as he has done for the world of tennis, Peter brings his clarity of vision into the field of diet and exercise. A must read for anybody who is under stress."

Peter G. Hanson, M.D.
Author of *The Joy of Stress*

"If anyone is qualified to write a book on total health, it is Peter Burwash—athlete, philosopher, lover of life, and one of the healthiest people I've ever met. In these pages, Mr. Burwash presents a collection of "life lessons," ranging from nutrition to ecologically balanced living, with the wisdom and compassion of a

teacher who's "been there." This sage guidance on achieving total health is a gift for your body, for your spirit, and for the health of the entire planet."

Michael A. Klaper, M.D.
Director, Institute of Nutrition, Education and Research
Author, *Vegan Nutrition, Pure & Simple*

*"*Total Health *is a compelling guide to the importance of diet changes in health, along with practical advice for putting science to work for better health. Peter Burwash knows the science of nutrition, and blends his own perspective as one who has made his own journey and is able to share his wisdom."*

Neal D. Barnard, M.D.
President PCRM
(Physicians Committee for Responsible Medicine)

"Peter again serves an ace with Total Health. *He has been a role model for me for years, and this book exceeds even my lofty expectations. No one can fail to benefit from time spent with Peter Burwash's approach to life and* Total Health *is Peter."*

Howard F. Lyman, J.D.
President, International Vegetarian Union

Howard F. Lyman, a fourth-generation rancher, winner of the Peace Abby Award, has learned that no animal needs to die for him to live.

*"*Total Health *inspires and empowers the reader. Every compact morsel of information compels positive life change. Peter's words practically leap off the page. His book is a*

perfect choice for those who want to keep their health and life in balance."

Paul F. Wenner, Chief Creative Officer (CCO). Inventor of the Gardenburger™, Wholesome and Hearty Foods, Inc. Author of *GardenCuisine, Heal Yourself and the Planet through Lowfat, Meatless Eating*

"In sound bites, Peter dishes out information everyone striving to attain and maintain total health should know. He is tireless in his quest to bring everyone to a higher quality of life."

Kathy Hoshijo
Nutritional Consultant, Author, *Kathy Cooks Naturally*

"Peter Burwash's intense effort to improve health and increase the enjoyment of life of people all over the world has been expressed now in this new book. He writes in such a personal way that you feel almost as if you are getting a letter directly from Peter. Not only does he cover the scientific matter well, but he inspires you to dive in—the water is perfect. Reading Total Health *is like a visit to the doctor and attendance at an enjoyable seminar covering a large field of health—mental, physical, and emotional."*

Agatha M. Thrash, M.D.
Preventative Medicine

"The Total Health *message should appear on the label of everything we eat and drink! It is an eye-opening must read."*

John Douillard, D.C.
Author, *Mind Body and Sport*
Owner, LifeSpa, Rejuvenation through Ayur-Veda

Testimonials

"Peter Burwash has been a tremendous inspiration to me, my wife Patty, and many of my employees through his books, speeches, and especially through his personal example. There's no question that following Peter's guidelines for diet and fitness will result in a happier and healthier lifestyle for anyone."

Rob Thibault
Owner/President, TS Restaurants of Hawaii and California

"Peter Burwash's message was an invaluable stepping stone to the attitudinal principles that has not only helped us optimize our health, but has helped us realize successes in other areas of our lives. Thank you, Peter! If you're looking for a healthier and happier life, this book is a must!"

Victor and Myra Brandt
Hawaii

"We were first introduced to Peter Burwash's concept of vegetarianism at a conference in Maui in 1992. His stimulating presentation prompted us to try going meatless for one week. Our one week trial extended to two, then three, then four weeks. We were feeling great—more energy, no afternoon blahs, etc. It has been five years since we decided to go meatless for a week. We are grateful to Peter for putting us on the right track to a more healthful lifestyle."

John and Linda Anderson
Hawaii

"One of my life's greatest discoveries was the message of vegetarianism by Peter Burwash. Amazing energy and superior health are a daily joy and life-long dream with increasing hope for the health of our planet."

Ron Estrada
Honolulu, Hawaii

"I was in my early twenties when I first heard Peter Burwash speak on being a vegetarian. It was one of the turning points of my life. Not only did my eating habits change, I began to see the world from a new perspective. I am now in my mid-thirties. I have traveled the globe and experienced greater success than I dreamed I would. The start on the road to change, growth, and fulfillment began with becoming a vegetarian."

Jeff Henkelman
Bali, Indonesia.

"We have been thinking of you almost every day since your visit to Blue River. Your presentation left a wonderful impression, and all the guests are noticing it. Now we are trying to maintain that image and service. Just for your information, numerous staff have not eaten any meat since your conference."

Mike Weigele
Blue River, Canada

Contents

Foreword

by

John Robbins

From every direction, it seems, more and more people are going veggie. They're making the vegetarian choice because they care about animals, or because they are concerned about the environment, or because they are taking the responsibility for their health, or because they are worried about world hunger. They are sick of being sick, and tired of feeling powerless. They are taking charge of their lives.

Some of us know why this crescendo is rising, why this movement toward a more compassionate, healthy, and environmentally sustainable way of eating is gathering increasing strength with every passing hour. There are few people more knowledgeable or sensitive to the historical importance of this development than Peter Burwash. Uniquely qualified to explain the factors that are involved in total health, he is one of the leaders of a movement whose time has come.

Not long ago the average American mother would have been more upset to learn that her son or daughter was becoming a vegetarian than to learn that he or she was taking up smoking. It was thought that you have to be a very special kind of person to be a vegetarian. It was seen as something on the fringe and offbeat. But today, thanks to Peter Burwash and others working alongside him, that has changed. Now we find even diehard meat eaters talking about eating less meat, or moving in a vegetarian direction. Not that long ago, people making vegetarian choices had to explain and justify themselves.

Today, the shoe is on the other foot. Now people who persist in eating meat increasingly feel a need to explain that they are cutting down.

And this is to the good. It's to the good for the health of all of us. It's to the good for the health of our rivers, topsoil, air, water, rainforests, and other biosystems. It's to the good for the animals whose lives are nightmares of suffering in the factory farms that have replaced yesterday's family farms.

Dear Reader, it's to your own good that you have picked up *Total Health* by Peter Burwash. Read it, and heed its wise and compassionate counsel, and you will be well on the way to a new level of aliveness, healing and joy.

John Robbins
Author, *Diet For A New America* and *Reclaiming Our Health*
Founder, EarthSave International

Introduction

Nothing in this book is intended to constitute medical treatment or advice. The primary goal of the book is to inspire a better understanding of your health, your body, and your environment. With that understanding you will be able to make a more informed choice for evolving changes in your lifestyle.

If you do decide to make broad changes in your lifestyle, it is advisable to have a medical physician or other health care practitioner as your partner in this transition. Fortunately, there are ever-increasing numbers of doctors placing prevention before cure in their medical practices.

Requests and an Apology

In preparing this book, it was not my intention to write a medical or health manual, but simply to address some very important issues. I am not a doctor or a scientist, just someone who has passionately and intensely studied the following material for over thirty years. Sure, I have a degree in physical and health education and also certifications in nutrition and exercise, but these academic excursions were minimal when compared to the practical knowledge gained from visiting 134 countries.

Whenever a book such as this is written, there is always some segment who will challenge the information, the statistics and research. To help ease the minds of skeptics, they should know this book took ten years to prepare and two years to write. The preparation involved visiting hospitals, meeting with doctors of all medical persuasions worldwide, visiting different cultures, and subscribing to and studying every medical health journal and book I could find.

In other books along this line, there are pages and pages of references. It is very easy to put a reference down, even if the information is incorrect. Also, I often have found that statistics are guesstimates. Therefore, whenever a statistic is quoted, I give a conservative number, unless I was able to get very specific data (in which case it will be referenced). I have avoided including product-sponsored research, since it is often biased.

Before progressing, I have three requests. The first is to trust the statistics. If there was any doubt (in my own mind), they were not included in the book. Secondly, please keep in mind that this book was written from a global perspective—a blend of East and West. Finally, as you begin to read, put your ancestral traditions and business interests aside. Look at the issues both personally and as a citizen and caretaker of the planet. I apologize in advance to those whose business plans may not be in "synch" with the thoughts and information in this book. Sometimes we get caught between our conscience and our pocketbooks. Yet remember, the most successful people and businesses in the world keep an open mind and adjust strategies as their sphere of knowledge expands—for, eventually, the impact of accelerated information will implement these positive changes for the planet and its peoples anyway.

The Journey of a Life-Shaping Experience

All of us have had one or more experiences in our lifetime that we can look back on and truly call "LIFE SHAPING EXPERIENCES." Unfortunately, many of these experiences are traumatic—we are shocked into reality or change. Reading a book can be a gentle or a forceful life-shaping experience. I hope this book has the influence of both those qualities.

In the past few decades, our world has broken apart at an alarming rate. The dramatic increase of heart attacks, cancer, and AIDS—coupled with an ecological devastation of the planet, as we continue to rape nature unabated—has forced us to reshape our consciousness, both personally and collectively. The Industrial Revolution began the destruction of a harmonious relationship between nature and human beings by teaching us to see nature as a commodity. I'm not so naive as to think that just one book can make much difference, but maybe a few seeds of thought and action will be planted in whomever might read it.

In 1970, I had a life-shaping experience that came as a result of a poorly thrown Frisbee. At the time, I was playing the professional tennis circuit and resting a few days in Hawaii before heading south for the New Zealand circuit. While tossing a Frisbee on Waikiki Beach, the Frisbee left my hand, headed to the right and kept spinning, until it dive-bombed onto the head of a gentleman peacefully enjoying the sunny day and blue water in front of him. I felt very bad and immediately ran over to apologize.

He was reasonably cordial, and we started talking. I learned that he was in Hawaii for a preventive medicine conference. When he found out I was a professional tennis player, he asked if I was aware that an athlete should not eat any meat, fish, poultry, or eggs six months before an event. I told him I wasn't interested in hearing that, since I loved my rare steak and roast beef. Besides, I had never eaten a salad before, and I felt that fruits and vegetables were for monkeys.

Despite my closed mind, he invited me along the next day. We shook hands and wished one another well. I had no intention of going to his seminar, as I felt great. Why I ended up going I can't recall. Perhaps deep down I wanted an edge over my fellow competitors. Perhaps I knew it might be interesting. (I had contemplated becoming a doctor at one time.) Perhaps it was just fate and I instinctively knew that everyone you meet is your teacher, if you are willing to be the student.

Whatever the reason, I walked out of that symposium with an understanding and a commitment to never eat meat, fish, poultry, or eggs again. This was a radical transition for me because I disliked most fruits, vegetables, and beans. It would be tough existing on French fries and spaghetti. But, as the doctors explained, my taste buds would change as I purified my body with quality foods. And ultimately they did, to the point where I now enjoy many dishes I have discovered only since that time.

I look back on that life-shaping experience as one of the most important in my life. Had I not unexpectedly met that doctor, there is no way I would have made the effort to visit a slaughterhouse—an experience which ultimately started me on the path to understanding and appreciating a deep reverence for life. Nor would I care what is going on with rain forests many thousands of miles away.

During my readings in that first year of transition, I remember a quote that is forever in the forefront of my thoughts: "Meat eating builds up a mentality of indifference." Looking back, this quote rings quite true to me. I really was very indifferent to the suffering of the world's animals and even its human population, what to speak of the more insidious global destruction taking place. And so I have to be grateful that my poor Frisbee toss—I'd like to blame the wind—resulted in a flight of discovery.

Without one's health, there is little one can truly enjoy. And once time heals, we forget our past illness and our terrible misery. The next time you are sick and lying in bed, go through a list of things you feel like doing. It will be a very short list.

You can and should be the architect of your health. Nutrition is the foundation of our physical well-being, followed closely by exercise and a good attitude. After observing people for many years attempting to change their lifestyles, I've learned that so much revolves around an understanding and commitment.

For example, almost one-half of the adult population in the U.S. is constantly trying to lose weight, yearly spending over thirty billion dollars. Many work extremely hard but with little results. Or once they get to their desired weight, they see this as a liberty to return to their old habits. It is estimated that only two to five percent of those who attain their desired weight goals or inch loss actually stay there. And there is a high percentage who quit before even reaching their goal. Some quit even after the first day.

For those who quit smoking, perhaps the toughest addiction of all, their goal was accomplished first by understanding what smoking was doing to their health and, secondly, by becoming committed. It may have been a simple commitment to stop because the smokers didn't like the taste in their mouth in the morning. Or it may have been a commitment to their children, who wanted them to attend their college graduation—something in doubt if they continued to smoke.

Nutrition and exercise go hand in hand. For years it was believed, if you exercised, it didn't matter what you ate. However, it is becoming increasingly clear proper nutrition is the crown jewel of all health. This has to be your foundation. This book will focus a lot on nutrition, but not just from a physiological point of view. I have found that those who understand nutrition from a moral and ecological perspective almost always keep their commitment. If an individual changes their nutritional lifestyle for personal

7

health reasons only, it's a rare person who won't cheat now and then.

Over the years of conducting seminars, there are always people in the audience who will say, "But everything in moderation." This phrase was the most frustrating to answer because it was an opinion instead of fact. One night an answer arrived. I said to the gentleman, "Moderation is half way between disaster and discipline." I am not sure of the origin of this phrase, but it was probably the result of two instances that day. The first was a visit to an alcoholic ward in a hospital. In talking with patients, I learned that each one of them had been a moderate drinker at one time. The second stemmed from a book I had been reading on discipline. It disclosed the fact that without discipline in your life and your habits, there will always be chaos. And with discipline, you can become free, contrary to the liberal thinking so prevalent in the 1960s and 70s. In both our personal and professional lives, we are coming to realize the importance of having discipline, even though the word itself has an aura of deprivation. BESIDES, WITH NUTRITION, MODERATION CAN GIVE YOU HEART DISEASE.

In addition to helping you understand so you can become more committed, I have tried in this book to help demystify the medical world. If you have ever listened to a doctor lecture, it is very easy to become lost in an ocean of medical terms—fats are lipids, heart attacks are myocardial infarctions. There is a limited use of medical terms in this book, so you can learn as you read without having to regularly refer to a dictionary or glossary at the back of a book.

In presenting a new lifestyle, the biggest challenge comes from those whose addiction to a particular food is entrenched or those whose incomes depend on the sale of a particular product. When John Robbins came out with his book, *Diet for a New America,* the meat industry was very upset. It is interesting how they have controlled the airwaves, propagating their so-called "healthy" food through advertising. Yet when someone exposed the atrocities and deception that were going on in their industry, they became very agitated. They had good reason though, because that one book reshaped a lot of people's lifestyles and thinking. And the more upset the meat industry became, the more books were sold. If the mainstream media exercises their editorial freedom to promote vegetarianism, the meat industry will often retaliate by threatening to cut off advertising dollars.

In the name of progress, these last few decades have moved at such a dizzying pace that, up until now, only a limited number of people have taken the time to understand and attempt to change the course of their personal destruction. Instead of a lifestyle that so many people have sought, they have created more of a death-style. We have adopted a lifestyle that harms us instead of keeping us healthy.

All of us at some point have made a difference in someone else's life. A major goal of this book is to help you become healthier so you can make a difference in many lives—your immediate family, your friends, animals, or even those tribes in the rain forest whose knowledge of the land and medicinal cures dwarfs that of even the best scientists and doctors. Who knows, by your caring about their welfare and helping to keep their lifestyle intact, they may some day return the favor to you with a cure that will help save a loved one. The longer we live, the more we realize that life does come full circle—it just takes time.

The Commercialization
of Our Life

Most of modern society now has an enormous addiction to food that is extremely unhealthy. But more importantly, in order to supply us with this unhealthy food, we are doing untold irreparable damage to our planet. A dedication to materialism and instant personal gratification has put us on a collision course with our environment. The consumer mentality of the past few decades has resulted in a highly commercialized, depersonalized society. We have to rethink our lifestyles. Changing it may not be a choice; it may be the only choice.

We are running faster and faster to stay on the treadmill of modern-day life. We have moved rapidly in our transition from a farm-oriented society to an industrialized society. We are losing millions of acres of farmland to erosion and development. We have lost our connection to nature and our land to the point that kids today think hamburgers grow on trees. Our alienation with nature is destroying our humanity.

Sophisticated marketing campaigns, coupled with a lack of good nutritional education in the schools, mean that unhealthy and undesirable eating habits are established early in life. Children are overpowered by commercials on TV, and as adults we remain trapped in a cocoon of believing that there is a fix-it pill or drug for all of our ills. Less than three percent of the ads on TV are for nourishing foods. The manufacturers of these unhealthy foods don't care what shape your arteries and heart are in.

13

U.S. business policies and the personal consumer choices of its people affect what goes on in the world, both directly and indirectly, when it comes to an emerging commercial global lifestyle. The rest of the world copies the "good" and the "bad" of American culture. Under the "bad" falls the dietary habits of the American population. U.S. exports of the fast-food mentality are probably the greatest disservice we could perform. Most of our children are living on "instant junk," and we are channeling these eating programs to other nations' children. Armed with huge advertising budgets and an aggressive marketing strategy, inroads into all the world's peoples' pockets are being made to quickly establish addictions.

In a survey of Japanese boys and girls, it was found that the girls' top two food choices were hamburgers and ice cream; the boys opted for pork and ice cream. As Japanese teenage girls continue to increase their dependence on the Western diet, the onset of their menstrual cycle begins earlier and earlier, just like their American counterparts. In the past one hundred years, the onset of the American female's cycle has gone from 17 1/2 years of age to 10 1/2 years of age. The onset of a girl's menstrual cycle in most Asian and African countries occurs in the late teens. An earlier cycle means an earlier desire and capability to bear children. Physiologically they may be ready, but otherwise they are not. The only difference in lifestyle is in their eating habits.

Japanese adults who convert to a Western diet suffer coronary disease at the same rate as Americans after only a few years. The fat, balding Asian male was a rarity until the recent introduction of the fat-laden, hormone-laced, standard American diet. The hormones injected into modern foods are not on any labels—and they won't be for a long time.

Food is America's biggest business. And the fast-food chains' demands have become the farmers' commands. The main concern of major food conglomerates is profit, not health. The seeming current interest in health is nothing more than another marketing ploy.

2.1 Slaughterhouses and Factory Farms

The lamb's body trembled with fear, a fear her predecessors in the long line had conveyed to her by their horrific screams. I stood no more than six feet away and looked into those eyes. Terror was tattooed on her eyeballs. It was a helpless feeling as the gun was placed beside her head. The trigger pulled. Within a second, her four trembling legs buckled. Her body lay in a heap, to be whisked away, carved and packaged for a grocery store hundreds of miles away.

My feeling of helplessness was quickly transformed into anger and disappointment. The anger was for the terrible injustice taking place behind four windowless walls with so few people aware of this hellish environment. If one wanted a glimpse of what hell might be like, a trip to a slaughterhouse is probably a pretty accurate review. My feeling of disappointment was with myself—that I could have lived twenty-five years being so utterly ignorant and blind to what was going on.

I had decided to go to a slaughterhouse, not because it was on my top-ten wish list, but because I wanted to reinforce my commitment not to eat meat anymore. I was convinced, from a health point of view, that abandoning my addiction to those rare steaks and Sunday roast beef dinners was in my best interest. Yet, I knew it would be very easy to cheat if I ate solely from a selfish point of view. Many people rationalize an occasional hamburger with a self-absorbed statement like, "A little piece of meat isn't going to hurt me." How selfish! Does that little piece of meat come without any suffering to another creature? When we look at the larger picture and transgress our own sense of gratification, we can always become more committed.

The picture of that lamb and the look in her eyes were my commitment. As her limp body was moved from the spot where her life force was taken from her, I said to her, hoping that she might somehow still hear and understand, "I'm sorry. I had no idea. I will never support this horrendous enterprise again."

Even in our worst nightmares, we don't see the brutalities which take place in a slaughterhouse. For the noble cow, the final horror begins on the trip to the slaughterhouse when they are packed tightly into transportation trucks for a trip that can legally last up to thirty-six hours in America. Tired, thirsty, and often sick after such an uncomfortable, stressful journey on their last ride, these beautiful, sentient creatures are unloaded and herded into holding pens. In some slaughterhouses, the horns are knocked off to allow for tighter confinement in the pens. Some animals are dead after the trip; this is calculated into the cost of doing business. Those downed animals who didn't survive are sometimes sent through the processing plants, ending up on our plates or in canned pet food.

Anyone who has watched the animals in a holding pen can see the terror in their eyes. By smelling and hearing those inside, they know their fate. They are aware that the walk up the chute will be their last one and there is absolutely nothing they can do about it. The livestock industry has become so depersonalized that these innocent animals are viewed simply as "products." Yet, these animals are living, breathing creatures who have a right to live. All beings resist death in their own fashion. They all tremble beforehand and scramble for their lives.

When the time arrives for them to be forced up the chute, they react in sheer terror. They watch those in front of them bellow loudly. Their next step is when they are stunned by a blank cartridge or sledgehammer and sink to their knees. Bullets are not used so that the brain can be salvaged for human consumption. The animal, still alive, is then hoisted up by its hind legs. Its throat is cut with a long knife and, at some point, it bleeds to death. The transition from living creature to cellophane-packaged meat has begun. The carcass is then dehided, split, and weighed. The speed with which the animal is dismembered is amazing. The disassembly line ensures that every part of the animal is used for food or an industrial purpose. This careful usage of all body parts has nothing to do with an ecologically sensitive industry but, rather, a greed to maximize profits.

The kill floor is characterized by suffocating smells and deafening screams. The screaming of the panic-stricken creatures is so loud that workers often wear ear protection. The condition of the workers is extremely hazardous. The floor is a red sea of blood and is treacherously slippery. The workers, covered with animal fat buildup, wear hip boots and blood-splattered coats while working at such a dizzying rate it is no wonder the industry has both a very high injury rate and the highest turnover rate of any job. In the typical slaughterhouse, three hundred animals are killed per hour.

Although there are a lot of people working,

there aren't any smiles. When I interviewed these people, I found that not one of them liked the job. In fact, many of them were terribly remorseful and suffered emotional trauma about what they were doing. I got the feeling that, even though this violent world of the slaughterhouse was legal and certified, deep down they all knew what they were doing was wrong. It just didn't feel right, not only on the floor but off the floor, but personnel are under strict orders not to speak to the press.

As our society becomes more and more violent, perhaps the echoes of past sages, philosophers, and spiritual teachers will ring more clearly: "If we come to respect the life of an animal, our respect for human beings will increase proportionately." The ghastly carnage of a slaughterhouse, where perfectly innocent creatures feel betrayed by us, is perhaps the most important sign of a society gone astray.

We put violence behind closed doors so we can ultimately feast our eyes on a "beautiful buffet" of sliced pieces of meat.

But just as injustices before have been uncovered, the time has also come where we shall become sensitive to perhaps the greatest injustice—on the outskirts of our cities, twenty million animals are slaughtered daily in the U.S. alone. Learning to respect life is one of the greatest lessons we can learn. The next time we go shopping and don't stop to pick up those cellophane packages of meat, we are saying that we now understand what is going on behind those closed doors.

The Western world was the first society to treat meat as a staple; and in order to satisfy the consumer demand, the factory farm was born. Factory farms are animal concentration camps—intense confinement systems, void of even a semblance of natural life. Farm animals

23

no longer live the idyllic life portrayed in nursery rhymes, and the owners of factory farms are not affectionate caretakers of animals. Most of the meat and chicken eaten today in the Western world comes from factory farms. Very, very few live in a free-range existence. Factory farms are a phenomena that really took off in the 1950s. These concentration camps were created primarily to maximize profits. The health and comfort of the animal is secondary. In fact, probably the unhealthiest creatures on the planet are factory farm animals, because of the horrid and unnatural conditions most are forced to endure.

If you cannot visualize what it is like for the animal, picture yourself having to live the rest of your life in a crowded elevator. The animal's entire life is a nightmare. Within days of their birth, life becomes a constant ordeal. Factory farm animals are squeezed to their biological limits. The pursuit of profit has resulted in living creatures being viewed as nothing more than robot-like biological machines. They are denied their basic instincts, and ultimately their lives.

Factory farms are not only debilitating for the animal, but virtually do nothing for society or our ecology. They are also a poor source of jobs. For example, one building having about 90,000 chickens requires only a few employees to oversee the operation. And the number of inspectors at the processing plants continues to decrease. And decreased inspectors will result in more diseases.

Because of the tight confinement of animals, disease is easily spread among them. So, antibiotics are introduced. Today, more antibiotics are used by farmers than by doctors. And this has major ramifications. Before a meat-eating person even tries a certain antibiotic, he may already have built up an immunity to it.

With profit as the motive, it is important to "turn over your inventory." Factory farms want to induce growth so they can fatten their animals up sooner and sell them. What is the solution? Hormones. The widespread use of antibiotics, hormones, and other drugs to offset disease-promoting conditions, as well as boost production, is prevalent in the Western world. And who is the ultimate recipient of these drugs? Is it any wonder our bodies are so toxic?

Ecologically, factory farms are devastating. The enormous amount of excess manure pollutes our ground, water, rivers, and lakes. Water is one of the critical staples of our diet, and we are allowing it to be contaminated on a daily basis in a major way that is totally unnecessary to our well-being.

Factory farms are improving in some countries such as Sweden, Switzerland, and Holland. The battery cages for laying hens are being abolished. But there is a long way to go, particularly in

America, which is the most backward as far as treatment of livestock is concerned. If we were to visit a factory farm just before we consumed the animals, only the most callous human-being would be able to eat.

In all of us, there is an inner compass that guides us. In even the most hardened of humans, there is a sensitive spark. Never was this more evident than in October of 1990 when a horse named Go For Win, racing at Belmont Park, fell and broke his leg. Since a horse's leg cannot be repaired, the tradition is to kill the animal. As Go For Win was shot, pictures were transmitted around the world showing robust, grown men in business suits with their compassionate wives and children crying unashamedly over the loss of this one creature. Yet, very few tears are shed over the millions of beautiful creatures that are living a life of horror in today's factory farms and dying daily in slaughterhouses.

2.2   Processed Foods

Another result of our commercially driven society is processed foods. Most of our food is industrially prepared. America leads the world in junk food consumption. We have gotten into the habit of altering almost everything we eat from its original state.

Packaged, processed food debuted in the 1920s, and the consumer society as we know it today was born. In the late 1930s, there were about 800 packaged items on grocery store shelves; whereas sixty years later, the number is around 10,000. In 1991, forty-four new products per day found their way onto grocery store shelves in the U.S. (*Vegetarian Times,* August 1992).

Processed food is actually destroyed food. Refinement robs our food of almost everything that is of nutritive value. The food is altered and devitalized. Nearly every vital element is removed, eliminated, or destroyed. It is laden with salts, sugars, preservatives, flavorings, and stabilizers. Just look at the lengthy list on labels.

We are selling poisonous products disguised as consumer products. It is a nutritional nightmare. Yet processed foods are convenient. And our selection of food today is determined by convenience and availability. Processed foods save us time . . . short term. We get our food on the table quicker; but long term, these processed foods erode our health. Dr. Denis Burkitt, who from 1946–1966 spent twenty years as a missionary doctor in Uganda, points out that we have altered our diet more in the last 150 years than throughout the entire course of civilization.

We need to shift from refined to unrefined foods. The availability of processed, refined foods has reduced our consumption of natural sources of nutrition. It is important, however, not to be fooled by the word "natural" on labels. "Natural" means coming from nature—no matter how far removed and refined the end product is. We should learn to read labels better and be suspicious of any food that has to be colored.

Understanding what a process like the hydrogenation of fats (used primarily for preservation) does is important. This process adds a hydrogen molecule to the fat molecule to keep it from becoming rancid by making the fat very stable so it won't spoil. The problem is that the body has a very difficult time breaking down such treated fat. These hydrogenated fats slow down the liver's ability to excrete cholesterol, allowing cholesterol levels in the blood to rise dangerously, and thus probably playing a significant role in atherosclerotic plaques clogging the arteries.

And what about the mounds of salt poured into our processed foods? Salt is very valuable to the industry, as it masks the bad odors of spoiled foods. We need to insist on tougher labeling laws. For example, fast-food chains are not required by law to reveal what is in the food they serve. And with the 160,000 fast-food outlets and the 583,000 food service outlets in the U.S., there is a lot of food being served to people who have no idea what they are really eating.

We need to realize that WHAT WE EAT is the single largest influence upon our bodies. The number one priority for any food should be its nutritional value. What we eat either nourishes or depletes our cells and organs, and affects our entire system. Food is the fuel that drives our body. Scientists are slowly revealing that the food we eat affects the body like a powerful dose of medicine. Food choices do matter.

We need to take time to become better informed about our health. We cannot swallow every commercial that comes our way. We would do well to follow an old Spanish proverb which

31

says, "A man too busy to take care of his health is like a man too busy to take care of his tools."

We need to take time to appreciate our food. Food should be eaten with a prayer of gratitude. How often is it that we sit down to a table, and within seconds of the food being placed on the table, we have a fork-full of it in our mouths? Why can't we just take a moment to say thanks for our meal? Fast food restaurants have disrupted the very important area of communication at mealtime. Today, we are not psychologically nourished. Before the 20th century, mealtime was for conversation, appreciation, and family. Today, twenty-five percent of Americans eat breakfast in their cars.

The capacity to abuse our body is greater than before. Most Westerners do not know what it feels like to be fully alert. Rich foods, transported long distances in throw-away packages, are not the answer for a quality life.

2.3   Attitudes Create Realities

The commercialization of our lives affects not only our food options, but also our emotional and psychological well-being. We are witnessing a revival of the understanding that our thoughts greatly affect our health. Many cultures have known the correlation between a pure mind and a pure body. The brain is part of the immune system. We have all known someone who, when asked how they are doing, always responds with some complaint. And guess what? They spend a good portion of their life in ill health. Whereas people who respond with "I'm doing great," even when they are sick, spend most of their lives in a healthy state. Thinking positive isn't just a cliché. It's good for the quality of our health.

Advertisements everywhere promise us a better life. They make us want more. They make us forget about what we have, and they put us in a state of anxiety. Should we buy it? Can we afford to buy it? TV commercials shape a child's concept of life, and the child carries this into adulthood. One hundred years ago, Americans spent about sixty percent of their income on food. Today, it is about fifteen percent. We buy more and more material goods. Then we have to insure it in case it is stolen.

If we are to obtain more, we have to work more. Then both spouses go to work. Our lives are rushed, and there is less time to prepare food. Fax this; Fedex that. Jobs are being eliminated, so you'd better not take a long vacation to re-create. And don't forget to stay in touch with the office while you're away. So when do we de-stress? When do we give our bodies a chance to relax, to rejuvenate, to repair? Stress breaks down our immune system and makes us more vulnerable to disease.

At the opposite end of the scale, there are

those who don't have anything to do. Being bored is just as stressful as being overworked. Very few of us today, busy or bored, take the time to watch a sunrise or a sunset.

2.4 Exercise

With such little spare time in our fast-paced lives and with little extra energy left, exercise is something that gets pushed to the back burner. We know we should exercise, but it is so much easier to be in charge of the remote control for the TV. One hundred and fifty years ago, at least fifty perecent of the population got enough exercise each day because of the physical work they did. Today, it is less than two percent. Our increasingly sedentary lifestyle has been made possible by technology. Elisha Otis, the inventor of the elevator, and Henry Ford have both indirectly

35

contributed to an increase in fat thighs and large stomachs.

Our brains may be on overload with the advent of the "information age," but our bodies are crying out for exercise. Our bodies are built to move. The heart is one hundred percent muscle, and a muscle that isn't exercised ends up atrophying. We have too much equipment designed to make life easier available to us now.

Our affluence has made lack of exercise and fatty diets a common way of life. Most of the diseases that ring up our health care bill are diseases we would not have contracted had we just eaten the right foods and exercised. Only after an untold number of people started dying of cancer, heart attacks, and other diet-related disease did the general population start to challenge the direction they were going.

Understanding Your Doctor
(And Modern Medicine)

When we get sick today, our approach seems to be to hand the problem over to someone else. When we were younger, we let Mom take charge. As we get older, we turn to our doctors. In addition, we blame something else for our ills. When we get a cold, we say it was caused by a draft or a family member. We seldom take personal responsibility for our illnesses or our cures.

Modern people seem to eat themselves into a diseased state and then undergo surgery. It's much easier to land ourselves in the doctor's office after significantly abusing our body and say, "Okay, Doc, fix me up." People with the coffee and doughnut lifestyle go to the doctor, get treatment, and return to their old habits. This is why one-third of what we eat today keeps us alive and the other two-thirds keep the doctors alive.

With the public crying out about health care costs, doctors are very much in the firing line. People are starting to realize that modern medicine, with its emphasis on cure rather than prevention, has a very high price tag, both short term and long term. The modern-day physician has become a repairman, and repairmen are expensive. As wonderful as modern medicine is in some areas, it's not getting us into better health. It is very easy to blame the medical profession, but we need to dig a little deeper to understand the real problems. Doctors are only human and tend to stick with what they know and have been taught. To comprehend the full issue, we need to look at the medical business and the medical schools.

Medicine is America's single biggest business. It is a sickness business. The sicker you are, the more money the doctor makes. The more people who are sick and/or are in need of surgery, the more money there is to be made. Doctors, hospitals, insurance companies, and pharmaceutical companies depend on sick people for their livelihood. Preventive medicine does not generate a lot of money. The incentives are all wrong. Even most insurance companies support the current system. If a heart specialist performs open heart surgery at a cost of $35,000, he or she is reimbursed by the insurance company with little or no questions. Yet, if the doctor spends half an hour talking about lifestyle changes that will begin to reverse the artherosclerotic build-up and prevent the need for surgery, the $50–$100 visit is usually not covered. The medical community has little incentive to emphasize prevention over treatment.

The U.S. has more hospitals and doctors than any country in the world, yet, as it builds more hospitals, there are more diseases. Modern medicine applies a lot of band-aids by treating the symptoms of disease, rather than studying and understanding real causes. But is this the doctors' fault? Do they have the knowledge? Do they want to become doctors of prevention? They have watched what happened to the dental profession, whose focus was on prevention. It meant less dental schools, less jobs, less patients. The doctors have a great thing going. Why change?

From a business perspective, they probably shouldn't change. But from a moral perspective, they have to change. Most doctors got into the profession because there was a space in their heart for caring, and many are committed to doing a truly great job. Yet, in modern medicine, doctors are seeing themselves fail. There is a growing number of doctors who, because they were truly frustrated, have voluntarily taken the preventive medicine path. But the change will have to come from within, because medical schools will be very slow to change.

In the medical schools, doctors are trained to treat disease, not prevent it. They are trained to deal with the patient after they have the problem. They are taught to suppress symptoms through drugs and surgery. Prescribing drugs and performing surgery are highly profitable for doctors, hospitals, and pharmaceutical companies. Despite an overwhelming amount of literature on nutrition and how it affects us, the average doctor receives about three hours of nutritional training in four years of medical school. The reason? Until recently, human nutrition had not been considered responsible for causing specific diseases, except in cases involving a lack of essential nutrients. Few physicians have even an elementary understanding of nutrition.

The most neglected question from your doctor is: "What do you eat?" In your last checkup, were you asked about your diet, your exercise program, and your lifestyle habits? Only a few doctors recognize the need for patients to change the overload on their digestive and immune systems. Some doctors think they are doing you a favor by labeling what your problem is as a particular disease. The time has come for the medical profession to focus not just on symptoms, but to also learn what the underlying causes are. They should start to put patients in charge of their health by teaching them how to eat right and exercise more.

For many doctors this will involve a personal lifestyle change as well. We have been getting a lot of advice from doctors who have not seen the inside of a gym for years. I remember staying at a resort in Fiji a few years ago, where there was a convention for Australian doctors taking place. While I was waiting for a taxi, a busload of doctors returned from an excursion. Coming off that bus were the most unhealthy, out-of-shape group of citizens one could imagine.

Personally, I think preventive medicine would be a big boost to doctors' personal lives as well. Healthier patients will mean fewer germs and diseases entering their offices. As Dr. John Sarno, author of *Mind Over Back Pain,* aptly put it, "Physicians should facilitate patient awareness and the utilization of nature's self-restoration process, releasing the potential within individuals to heal themselves."

Twenty-five hundred years ago, on the island of Cos, Greece, the purported founder of modern medicine, Hippocrates, sent a couple of important messages: "Thy food will be thy remedy." and "Everyone has a doctor in him. We just need to help him in his work." We have strayed from Hippocrates' guiding words with our current dependence on surgery and drugs and have become indoctrinated to believe such drastic invasiveness is normal.

Dr. Dean Ornish, assistant professor of medicine at the University of California at San Francisco College of Medicine, and who has authored a book on reversing heart disease, wrote, "I don't understand why asking people to eat a well-balanced, vegetarian diet is considered drastic while it is medically conservative to split people's chests open for surgery, have the veins in their legs plugged into their hearts, and put them on powerful, cholesterol-lowering drugs for the rest of their lives."

Most doctors offer only surgery or drugs as a cure, even though they know that one operation usually leads to another and that all drugs have side effects. Modern medicine performs far too many surgeries and over-prescribes drugs. A lot of today's medicine is an insult to the body. It has left a lot of people alive, but not well. There is no question, however, that there are some outstanding aspects of modern medicine. The real problem lies in the reluctance to slow down, or even take stock of, where the profession is headed.

Do we need to have such a dependence on prescription drugs? Our senior citizens are like walking pharmacies, averaging fifteen prescriptions per person. Almost fifty prescriptions are filled every second in the U.S., and 1.5 million people a year return to the hospital due to the side effects of drugs. Drug therapy is symptomatic therapy. Health cannot be purchased in a pharmacy. Yet, today's drug companies have infiltrated the medical profession through elaborate meetings, vacations, dinners, and courses sponsored by pharmaceutical companies to win doctors' loyalties. In 1985, doctors began selling drugs, even though they basically had a very limited knowledge of how the drugs were developed or what their long-term effects would be. Free samples and persistent salesmanship induce doctors to experiment on their patients with new drug therapies.

Today's patient feels very rushed. As a result of a tennis injury to my back in 1984, I spent ten years visiting doctors around the world. In the U.S. and Canada, the average time each doctor gave me was six minutes, and I felt like an intruder in their offices. Even though I told them I didn't believe in taking drugs, every one of them prescribed drugs for me. Not one doctor touched me, except to tap my knee or check my heartbeat. They didn't want to know what movements I could or could not perform.

They couldn't take the time to find out what the real problem was, but they all found the time to write a prescription. I ended up with a box full of unused drugs and a still painful back.

The doctor of the future must become more humble. They are treated as gods in our society, when instead they should be the consummate servants and teachers. Fortunately, there are more doctors each day stepping forward to join the ranks of those who are studying and learning about what Hippocrates said in 431 BC.

Understanding Your Body

If we paid as much for our body as we did for our house, we would become a much better caretaker. But since it was a present from our parents and we didn't have to spend our hard-earned dollars to get it, we assault it with so many unhealthy foods that it is amazing some of us live as long as we do. However, today, far too many people are dying too soon of diseases over which they could have significant control. People feel victimized when they find out they have cancer or are shocked when they have a heart attack. Both of these are a result of what we eat with our forks, chopsticks, or hands.

One of the courses which should be introduced into all elementary and high schools is a course on understanding our body. As I said earlier, this book is not intended to be a medical journal, so the following will be a simplistic, quick overview of some key parts of our body and how it functions. Knowledge of your body can help enhance the quality of your life.

4.1   The Heart

Your heart is your power plant. There aren't adjectives powerful enough to describe it. Incredible and phenomenal are close, but this magnificent piece of human machinery is unparalleled in the world. It is not an organ per se, but rather a muscle (100% muscle) about the size of the human fist with an average weight of nine and a half ounces (an obese heart weighs about thirteen ounces). The heart valves are as thin as tissue paper (about a few hundredths of an inch), yet they are sturdier than iron. The heart pumps blood to the lungs where it picks up oxygen. This oxygenated blood returns to the heart and then heads off to the rest of the body. The heart has enormous reserve power and pumps thirteen tons of blood every twenty-four hours.

The average heart rate in the U.S. for men is 72 and for women, 78. This is an average—a much too high average. Your goal should be a lower heart rate. An unfit heart has to beat ten to fifteen times more than a fit heart just to maintain body functions. In one day, this could mean 50,000 beats more than a conditioned heart. (In one year, that's 17 million extra beats.) The heart muscle can deteriorate without pain, as there aren't any nerves in the arteries to detect damage. Hence, the first sign of a heart attack can be sudden death.

4.2 The Blood: Our River of Life

We cannot have a healthy body without clean blood. Blood is our river of life. It bathes every cell in our body. The cells extract the nutrients they require from the blood. The bloodstream plays a healthy role in cleaning out our system. It is also the pathway for the body's toxins. When our doctor draws blood, it is for the purpose of locating certain foreign invaders. The bloodstream becomes helpless if it has to continuously assimilate toxins:

Blood cells have a natural propensity to repel one another. This allows them to flow smoothly and transport valuable oxygen to the cells. If cells don't get oxygen, they die. When fatty foods are eaten, sludging of the blood begins within one hour. The cells become coated and lose their natural repelling ability. With the cells sticking together (clotting), the heart has to work harder. After eating a cheeseburger, the blood becomes greasy with animal fat and stays that way for up to four hours. Poor circulation leads to malnourished, polluted cells and, as a result, poor organ function.

There is a normal amount of blood clotting that should potentially take place. If we are in a car accident and are bleeding internally, we need a valuable defense mechanism of blood clotting. It can be life-saving. Fish oil can prohibit clotting, yet this can work against the human being—as in the case of the Eskimos, who have the longest clotting time. Vikings talked about how easy it was to subdue the Eskimos because if they were cut, they would bleed uncontrollably. Their clotting time was around fourteen minutes—long enough to bleed to death. A good clotting time is three to seven minutes. A person on a vegetarian diet usually has the best natural clotting time of around three to four minutes. If you are going to have a blood test, wait at least twelve hours after eating. You will get a more accurate count.

4.3   Arteries

The body has 60,000 miles of blood vessels. Our arteries are like miniature water pipes and are responsible for delivering blood to the cells, while the veins return it. To put this in perspective, if you strung all of your circulatory system together, it would stretch around the world two times. And some people say this enormously complex body happened by chance.

4.4   Cholesterol

Up until 1984, only a small percentage of the population really knew or understood what cholesterol was. Although there is a greater awareness of cholesterol, most people still view cholesterol as bad. However, cholesterol is essential to life. It is a natural lubricant, indigenous to the body. It forms the building blocks of the outer membranes of our cells. Produced in the liver, it is found in all parts of the body. Eighty percent of blood cholesterol is produced in our body. It is not a fat but, rather, a type of sterol.

Cholesterol is produced in the liver of all animals. All animal products, with the exception of egg whites, contain cholesterol. There is no cholesterol in fruits, grains, vegetables, or legumes. Humans can excrete a limited amount of cholesterol (about 100 to 300 milligrams per day). Because of this slow, limited excretory capability, humans run into significant problems when they eat animal products. The average American is ingesting 500–600 milligrams of cholesterol per day, thereby banking hundreds of milligrams in their arteries daily.

There are two types of cholesterol, which have been in the news a lot in the past decade: HDL and LDL. LDL cholesterol tends to stick to the insides of the arteries like mineral deposits in a water pipe. HDL cholesterol, on the other hand, has a flushing effect. Think of HD as Highly Desirable. The body makes all of the cholesterol it needs. It is the excessive amounts eaten by Western societies that lead to heart disease. (See Chapter 6 on heart disease.)

4.5   The Digestive System

Your digestive system is your loyal servant. Even though there is a never-ending flow of food coming down the conveyer belt, it serves you faithfully. Digestion requires energy. In other words, food takes energy from the body before it can become a source of energy. It uses roughly thirty-three percent of our energy—more than any other system in our body.

Digestion of food begins in the mouth, with saliva breaking down carbohydrates. Fruits are assimilated into the body the quickest because when they are ripe, they are pre-digested (broken down). The emptying time of the stomach is between one to six hours (average four hours). Exercise and fiber help speed up digestion, while stress, fats, and alcohol slow it down. In the stomach, foods are bathed in acids and enzymes. Some assimilation of nutrients into the bloodstream occurs in the stomach, but the majority takes place in the small intestine (about ninety percent). The small intestine has millions of tiny, organ-like suction cups called villi, which draw nourishment into the blood. The nutrients are then taken to the liver, where they are split up.

Foods rich in carbohydrates leave the stomach

first, followed by proteins and then fats. This is why if you have a fatty meal late at night, you are likely to have poor sleep. Your unfortunate digestive system had to work all night, using your body's energy; when, in fact, sleep should have been for the regeneration of energy.

At rest, the stomach is about the size of a closed fist. How much can it comfortably handle? If you were to take food and fill your two cupped hands, it would fill about two-thirds of your stomach. When you see the volume of food some people consume, is it any wonder they have stomach pains after eating? It takes twenty to thirty minutes from the time we start eating for the brain to register that your stomach is full (satiety signal). You can eat an enormous amount in twenty to thirty minutes.

As we get older, many of us find we cannot digest (or handle) the vast quantities of food we ate when younger. Any big meal will deflate your mental acuity and energy; however, fat-laden meals, which are the slowest to digest, are definitely the worst.

4.6 The Colon: Your Trash Compactor

Your colon (large intestine) is a five-to-six-foot-long trash compactor. A clean colon is the best health insurance you can have. The colon is your sewage system. Its contents (stool) are made up of undigested food, fiber, water, and billions of bacteria. Stool is a highly adaptable medium for the prolific breeding of germs, bacteria, and viruses. Therefore, a short transit time in the colon is vital. You want to limit the exposure time that food is in contact with the bowel wall. Stools of meat eaters are much more compact and slow-moving than stools of vegetarians. Exercise also stimulates the colon.

The normal number of bowel movements

should correspond to the number of meals one eats—e.g., two meals a day, two bowel movements. At the least, one should pass solids once a day. The color of your stools should generally be light brown. They should be uniform, moderately soft, and easy to pass without pain or strain. You can often monitor your health by checking your stool—its regularity, color, and uniformity.

A vegetable-based diet—high in whole grains, fruits, vegetables, and other foods rich in complex carbohydrates—promotes regular bowel movements. The colon needs action, so fiber is very important. Fruits produce a looser stool. This is especially true of prunes, as they contain a chemical stimulant that has laxative-like effects. Plenty of water, drunk at least three hours after or thirty minutes before a meal, is also very conducive to proper digestion and elimination.

4.7 The Liver

The liver is the filter organ of the body. One of its principal purposes is to detoxify the body of foreign elements. The liver of all animals is responsible for chemical detoxification. It concentrates all pollutants consumed by the animal. Therefore, it is hard to understand why someone would want to eat an animal's filter system. The liver is responsible for almost five hundred separate functions in its role as the body's chemical factory and filtration plant. It can be overwhelmed by the accumulation of toxic substances, and when this happens, the toxins go into the bloodstream. When an overflow like this occurs, the person is likely to get sick. Alcohol is a poison and very toxic to the liver. Everybody should go to an autopsy to see the liver of a person who drank mostly water versus the scarred, contracted liver of a person who drank alcohol. You wouldn't need a medical degree to get the message.

The liver is the largest gland in the body, traversing eight to nine inches and weighing approximately four pounds. As food is digested and absorbed, the first stop is the liver. The liver dismantles it. The liver also produces bile, an enzyme that separates fat into small droplets. Without bile, fat cannot be broken down and properly absorbed.

Some cholesterol is made in the liver. If someone has a disease of the liver (cirrhosis, as in alcoholics), his or her cholesterol production will be lower. Therefore, a lower cholesterol count for an alcoholic may not be an accurate indicator of the health of the arteries.

4.8   The Kidneys

Kidneys are the masterpieces of biological

plumbing. They remove toxic waste, filtering the body's entire blood supply about twenty-five times a day. The kidneys are the final decision-maker as to what will be excreted. High protein diets are strongly associated with kidney disease, as the filtering units are destroyed by excessive exposure to protein. As with liver, people actually eat animals' kidneys. Kidney stew pie is a popular dish, yet why would anyone want to eat an animal's urine sac?

4.9 The Immune System: The Body's Police Force

The immune system is the body's police force. Its job is to protect the body from invaders that might infect you. It is your body's means of safeguarding your health. Your body is always striving for balance and a state of wellness. It is forever self-repairing, self-cleaning, and self-purifying—IF YOU GIVE IT A CHANCE. As Hippocrates said, "Everyone has a doctor in them." Your level of resistance ultimately determines how sick you will get. This is why some members of your family may seldom get sick, even though they are exposed to the same germs as everyone else in the family. They have a strong immune system.

Although almost every system in the body has some role in fostering immunity, a major share of the cleaning work is the responsibility of the immune system. Some of the medical terms related to the immune system, which may be familiar to you, are antibodies, macrophages, lymphocytes, phagocytes, white cells, etc. To simplify everything, your mobile police force, the antibodies, are like miniature PACMEN. They gobble up the invaders. Certain antibodies act like guided missiles. They attack specific germs. Your body secretes mucus to coat over an irritation. It's a method of entrapping potentially harmful substances. Your police force has three units: those on active duty, those on constant patrol, and those on reserve. They are attached to the walls, waiting for a call. For example, when you cut your finger, white blood cells travel to the area to help promote healing.

We need to learn to work in harmony with our immune system. When we have a cold, it is the body's natural protective mechanism to secrete mucus. Mucus is the first line of defense against millions of disease-causing bacteria trying to invade the body. And as the body gets rid of mucus, your running nose is the overflow. Yet, what do we do? We pump substances up our nose to stop the flow. Have you ever thought about where the mucus and toxins go? They go right back into your body to do more damage, prolonging your cold. If your body could handle the toxins internally in the first place, it wouldn't have tried to expel them externally.

The same goes for a fever. Fever is the body's way of keeping the virus from multiplying. It is an essential weapon in the body's response arsenal. It is best to let a fever run its course, unless you are in great discomfort or your temperature is above 103 degrees.

Something that your immune system would appreciate when you are ill is to stop eating for one to two days. I only incorporated this into my life style about ten years ago, yet I consider it one of the most important pieces of advice I ever received when it comes to health. It's common sense. The rest of the animal world instinctively knows this. Have you ever tried to get your dog or cat to eat when it was sick? No way. They do two things: stop eating and rest. When we stop eating, we allow our immune system (the "police force") to work at full capacity. Even if you eat healthy foods, you will always ingest foreign substances that put your immune system to work. Digestion requires a lot of energy; so, if you eat while sick, you'll overwork your body and, thus, delay your recovery.

Secondly, we should rest. This, too, allows your body to use its full resources to fight infection. After we exercise, our body tissues have to be repaired, a responsibility of the immune system. We have a lot more to learn from the animal world.

How do we keep our immune system strong? Probably the foremost approach is to eat the proper foods. (See Chapter 5.) We should only eat foods which will strengthen our immune system. In the news lately are many articles about free radicals and antioxidants. When cells are damaged, free radicals are produced. These are villains and can be neutralized by what are called antioxidants, a group of vitamins, minerals, and enzymes—especially vitamins C and E, beta-carotene, and the mineral, selenium—that protect the body from free radical damage.

Also prevalent lately are articles on psychoneuroimmunology, which is the power of the brain to heal the body. There is little doubt that the body's immunity is under the ultimate jurisdiction of the brain. The mind and immune system communicate with one another. The immune system is like a neon sign that flashes with your emotions. If they are positive, you are likely to be strong and healthy. If they are negative, your immune system gets clobbered. What goes on in your mind affects the chemical composition of cells in your body. In other words, the body is a reflection of the mind.

In addition to positive thoughts, humor can be very important. Studies have shown that people who use humor have more infection-

67

fighting antibodies. Everyone should have a friend who makes them laugh.

For babies, breast milk is best for a strong immune system. When a mother breast feeds, the first secretion before the milk is colostrum, which is rich in immune agents.

Exercise also plays a major role. The lymphatic system (where white cells reside) has thousands of miles of lymph vessels that parallel your circulatory system. The flow of the lymph fluids depends on the contraction of many muscles to push it through one-way valves (unlike the blood, which is pumped by the heart). Exercise gets the lymph flowing. Also, exercise elevates the body temperature. Like a fever, exercise increases the number of white cells in your blood.

It is extremely important to keep your cells healthy. It is difficult for any kind of germ or virus to attack clean, healthy cells. Unfortunately, however, most Westerners have chronically depressed immune systems and are constantly damaging and weakening their cells, leaving them very vulnerable to disease.

Here are some of the principal enemies of a strong, healthy immune system: caffeine, tobacco, alcohol, refined foods, chemotherapy, excess sugar, exhaustion, and stress. There is also strong evidence that dietary fat is another culprit.

A team of researchers in Heidelberg, Germany, began a study on the immune system in 1978. Recently, they found that the white blood cells of vegetarians had more than double the ability of their non-vegetarian counterparts to destroy cancer cells (*Vegetarian Times,* October 1991, Dr. Neal Barnard). Up until recently, the general feeling was that if we ate healthy meals, we didn't need to supplement them with vitamins and minerals. However, with the discovery of the effects that so many chemicals and radiation have on our bodies, we may need these extra vitamins and minerals to bolster our immune system; even more so to counteract the subtle, yet devastating, effects of our advanced technological world.

4.10   Toxins

A toxin is any substance which creates irritating and/or harmful effects on the body, undermining our health. A normally functioning body was created to handle a normal level of toxins. In the modern era, it is the overload that is hurting us. A sick body is a toxic body. The proper function is slowed in all body tissues in which toxins have settled. Sick (toxic) people are always tired people. As long as there is toxic waste in your system, a good portion of your available energy goes toward eliminating it.

Toxins are eliminated through your lower

intestine, bladder, lungs, and skin. One-third of our toxins are released through our skin. Yet, twenty-three billion dollars a year are spent in the U.S. alone on skin care lotions, many of which clog the pores and force the toxins back into the body.

.Nature gives us warnings that toxic poisons have built up in our bloodstream (headache, sore throat, white tongue, etc.). Toxins also build up in our joints and lymph nodes. All of us have stored toxins in our bodies. Poisons and toxins accumulate in the fatty tissues of all animals. Toxins and fat cells can be reduced by shedding extra pounds (an extra incentive to shrink your fat cells).

4.11 Bacteria

When people think of bacteria, they think of something bad. Yet without bacteria, all life

71

would cease. Good health depends on having a high percentage of friendly bacteria, as they feed on toxic waste within the body.

4.12   Enzymes: The Body's Labor Force

Enzymes are our body's labor force. They are the sustenance and essence of our lives.

Without enzymes, life is impossible. All organs, tissues, and cells are run by enzymes. They are at the heart of every chemical action in the body. They are the digestive catalysts, whose function is to break down the food we eat into a chemical structure that can pass through the membrane of the cells lining the digestive tract and then proceed to the bloodstream. This is a very important process, and each enzyme has its own specific job.

Enzymes only work within a limited temperature and are destroyed by excessive heat and cold. Heat above 116 degrees starts killing enzymes, rendering them useless. This is why it is always best to lightly steam your vegetables— enzymes are more abundant in raw, fresh food.

Enzymes are delicate and are an easy prey for foreign invaders. Just as there are many substances that can harm our immune system, enzymes also have their unwanted list: alcohol, tobacco, drugs, coffee, fluoride and chlorine in drinking water, additives, and preservatives. As well, refining, processing, and pasteurizing destroy enzymes—all the more reason to eat our food in its most natural state. Stress can also deplete the body's enzyme supply.

There are three types of enzymes, the first two of which are inherent to the body:

Digestive: These are first secreted in the mouth's saliva and in the upper part of the digestive tract. There are approximately 1,300 digestive enzymes identified to date.

Metabolic: Those whose workplace is in the blood, tissues and organs.

Food: Naturally found in raw, uncooked food.

As you can see, our body is made up of many vital, interrelated parts that work as a team. They want to work in harmony. We, as the managers of our own bodies, should strive very hard to maintain that harmony by only introducing good teammates.

Understanding Nutrition

What you eat adds up to the single largest and most important influence on your body's well-being. Nutrition is the foundation of your health. Up until recently, eating meat was a sign of prosperity. Eating only beans, grains, and vegetables was a sign of poverty and a lack of social standing. Couple this perception with a constant barrage of slick advertisements, and we have a society that eats what they think they should eat, rather than what their bodies are capable of handling.

Contrary to what we have been told, the human being is physiologically not built to eat meat. Sure, there are historical accounts of cavemen and their hunting exploits, but a lot of this is myth built on speculation. No question there have always been segments of the population that have been driven by the desire to eat animal flesh, just as there have always been people who have killed others, whether it be for food (cannibals) or the pursuit of more land. But that indicates a brute, uncivilized way of life.

For many in the world's population, however, they are not the least bit concerned about whether our body is capable of processing meat. They believe it is wrong morally. Ideally—and according to the vision and aspiration of all world religions—the Earth is a paradise lush with gardens and without violence among her creatures.

Even prior to the Industrial Revolution, a majority of the world's population ate a predominantly vegetarian diet. One of the principal reasons was that their religion did not permit anything other. All the original religions teach that it is wrong to willfully kill an animal to eat, unless for survival there is no other choice. You will suffer a reaction if you do. ("As you sow, so shall you reap," and the law of karma.) A wonderful book on this subject is *Diet for Transcendence* by Steven Rosen.

For many, the motivation to alter one's nutritional lifestyle is strictly related to personal well-being. Others change because of compassion for the animal world and/or the environment. Whatever the reason, we shall now look at the variety of food options we have.

5.1 Four Food Groups

Marion Nestle, Chair of the Nutrition Department at New York University, said it best: "The standard four food groups are based on American agricultural lobbies. We have an extremely powerful meat lobby." Never was this more evident than in 1991, when a new group of four was proposed: vegetables, fruits, grains, and legumes (beans). The meat lobby immediately went to work, and the end result was a triangle which still included meat.

There is no scientific evidence for the original four food groups introduced by the USDA in 1956. That chart had nothing to do with health. Unfortunately, many teachers and parents saw it as the bible of nutrition, and those fancy, four-color posters became part of our nutritional education. Even nutrition schools adopted these, despite evidence that most people who eat the old four food groups die earlier (Dr. Neal Barnard). One can get one hundred percent of the nutrients required by the body without eating meat, fish, poultry, or eggs.

5.2   "How Do I Get My Protein?"

Along with the old four food group charts (meat, dairy, grains, and produce), the greatest myth propagated was that the body was best served by getting a "complete protein." Meat contains all the essential amino acids, so people were duped into thinking this was the way to eat. It is important to realize, however, that the body cannot use pure protein such as meat, chicken, poultry, and fish directly. The protein has to be broken down. This extra step is not only taxing and aging to the body, but it is also unnecessary.

At almost every seminar I have given, one of the first questions asked is: "What about protein if you don't eat meat?" Let's dispel this myth. There is absolutely no need for pure protein per se, but rather a requirement for amino acids, which are the building blocks of protein. And every amino acid you need is in fruits, vegetables, and grains. Plant foods contain the same eight essential amino acids found in animal foods, they're just in differing amounts. So, if you are eating a diet based on whole plant foods and are getting a minimum number of calories, there is simply no way you can be lacking in protein. People don't die of protein deficiency; they die of malnutrition. Protein deficiency is so uncommon it is a non-issue.

The second myth is that you need to consume all your essential amino acids at one meal. (In other words, you must eat rice and beans together.) This lacks scientific evidence. The body has amino acid pools in the blood, lymph, and liver that store amino acids. If one amino acid is not eaten today, it is secreted to make an ideal balance tomorrow.

The third myth is that protein builds bigger muscles. If we put our common sense hat on for a moment, we can see how ridiculous this myth is. Saying that eating an animal's muscle (animal protein) will improve your muscle mass and make you stronger is analogous to saying that if you eat an animal's brain you will get smarter. You will get bigger, stronger muscles by exercising, not through eating. Yet, many people, particularly Americans, feel that reducing their consumption of animal-based protein will compromise their health and make them weaker.

In addition to strength, some people still think that protein gives energy. Protein does not produce energy—it uses it. Only as a last resort is protein used as an energy resource. The body prefers carbohydrates and fats for its fuel. Protein may be the chief building material of our bodies, but it is a poor source of immediate energy. Also, animal protein carries with it a very hefty price tag—artery-clogging saturated fat and cholesterol.

The final myth is that animal foods have protein of superior quality. Well, the quality of protein in plant foods is enough to grow a horse, an elephant, or hippopotamus. Enough said about these myths.

Proteins are the essential bricks and mortars of the body. The word protein comes from the Greek word *proteus,* meaning of first importance. They are needed to build every cell in the body and are responsible for growth. Yet by our early twenties, most of our physical growth is completed, so repair, replacement, and maintenance become the key issues. When we were young, we needed a little more protein, but nowhere near what we pour into our bodies today. People who eat a lot of protein almost always look older because it overtaxes the body's organs, promoting degeneration and aging.

Proteins are large molecules that are difficult

to break down into the necessary amino acids. Excess protein results in an enlargement of the kidneys and liver as they attempt to compensate and excrete the unusual amount of protein. An overabundance of protein results in an overload on the immune system. When the body breaks the pure protein down from the flesh, a powerful toxic material called uric acid is ultimately released. As mentioned earlier, unlike carnivores and omnivores, humans don't have the enzyme uricase to break flesh protein down. Uric acid is one of the reasons meat eaters have stronger body odors.

Also, a diet with concentrated protein causes calcium to be leached from bones. The sulfur-containing amino acids in protein have to be neutralized with calcium. Calcium is a chaser. And remember where most of our calcium is: in the bones (about 98%). It is interesting to note the high incidence of osteoporosis in protein-consuming societies. (See Chapter 6.)

Since the body has a limited capacity to store protein per se, it either gets rid of it or stores it. Protein left over after the body has done its housekeeping is converted to fat and sugar, and then stored. Therefore, excess protein builds fatter bodies, not bigger muscles. Just look at the countries in which protein is the big staple in the diet, and you will see that they are grossly overweight.

Hopefully, the above has laid to rest the myths about protein. A ground swell of misinformation has resulted in an obsession with protein. Even on a vegan diet (no meat, fish, poultry, eggs, or dairy products), one gets twice the amount of required protein. So relax, and remember that the reduction of protein in your diet will be one of the best things you can do for the quality of your health.

5.3   Carbohydrates

The bulk of the food you eat should be carbohydrates. Carbohydrates are your human petroleum. They are your most readily usable and preferred source of energy. Long maligned as fattening, they are actually the food to eat if you want to lose weight. What they are is filling—in effect, great hunger satisfiers.

There are two types of carbohydrates: simple (fruits) and complex (vegetables, grains, pasta, etc.). They are stored in muscles and the liver as glycogen and in blood as glucose. Whereas the body has an unlimited capacity to store fat, it can only store a limited amount of carbohydrates (about 1,500 calories). Therefore, you need to eat carbohydrates regularly.

Carbohydrates have many advantages that make them the preferred choice of nutritional intake. They are more easily digestible than fats and proteins and are, therefore, less taxing on the body. The sugar in carbohydrates is released slowly and readily, thereby giving you a sustained source of energy.

Carbohydrates are rarely stored as fat. The body can turn simple carbohydrates into blood sugar (glucose) almost immediately. This is why fruits are your best source of quick energy. Your brain and nerve tissues use only glucose. Carbohydrates also cause the brain to manufacture serotonin, a chemical linked to calmness and cheerfulness.

The best carbohydrates are unrefined. Refined carbohydrates are processed by removing the outer shell or bran layer containing the valuable fiber. Most snacks are refined carbohydrates. All animal flesh is devoid of carbohydrates. Carbohydrates in their whole form (that is, whole grains, whole beans, whole potatoes, whole fruits and vegetables, etc.) should always be the foundation for a lean, healthy diet.

5.4   Fats

The body's ability to store fat is a marvelous survival mechanism. Fat plays an important role in overall health. We need fat in our diet; but the Western world, particularly the U.S., has gone overboard. In 1925, about ten percent of our calories came from fat. Today, it is fast approaching fifty percent. Anything over ten to fifteen percent is going to tax your body, unless you are an athlete or someone with an extremely high capability of burning off fat. The body appears to need very little dietary fat, yet in the U.S. we put gobs of fat on almost everything.

87

An unfortunate aspect of fatty foods is that they are very addicting. Fat tastes so good, especially when laced with sugar. We like fats because they are what make our food taste and smell so rich. Fats have very little flavor by themselves; they are actually flavor activators. They greatly enhance the flavor of our food. This is why if we do not cook with fats, we need to learn to use herbs and spices. Otherwise, our food is very boring, and we return to our old habits.

There are two types of fat: saturated fat, which is solid at room temperature (meats, eggs); and unsaturated fat, which is liquid at room temperature (oils). Fats store energy. They are the most concentrated form of energy (two times that of carbohydrates). Also, our nerves, muscles, and organs must be cushioned by a normal amount of fat. And, finally, fat ensures that fat soluble vitamins such as A, D, E, and K are properly transported and utilized.

The problem we face today with fats is excess. We eat way too much fat. With the exception of infants up to age two, we need to watch our fat intake—particularly since we tend to consume a lot of commercially processed foods, many of which are forty to fifty percent fat.

Virtually any food of animal origin is high in saturated fats––the kind that raises cholesterol. The meat industry is extremely keen on keeping the public in the dark about fat content. A strong meat lobby has enabled them to get away with not labeling meat.

Fatty material lands like lead in your stomach, causing a sludging of the blood and subsequent fatigue. Fat causes the blood cells to stick together. This means oxygen cannot get to the muscles in full force and waste products cannot be carried away as quickly as they should. Animal fats are the strongest promoters of clotting. The day you stop eating animal fats is the day your blood starts thinning out.

5.5   Meats

If you spend the first half of your life giving money to the meat industry, you will most likely spend the second half of your life giving money to the medical industry. Humans have no physical need whatsoever to eat meat. People eat meat because their taste buds crave it, it is convenient, or it is a habit––a part of their culture. However, with all the information we now have, the only reason someone would continue to eat meat is because of an indifference to their personal health, to the suffering of animals, and to the environmental destruction caused by the meat industry. Or they just don't get it. The disadvantages of eating meat are so numerous that one of the most difficult challenges in writing this book was keeping this section to a reasonable length.

Meat sales in the U.S. peaked in 1971. The shattering of the myth that meat was the ultimate source of protein helped reduce meat consumption. However, the real turnaround came when almost everyone seemed to know someone personally who had suffered a heart attack or had cancer. The modern health crisis was in full swing, and people started changing their eating habits. One of the first items to be scratched from the meal plan was red meat. But there is still a long way to go, as atherosclerosis (clogged arteries to the heart or brain) is still, by far, the biggest killer in industrialized countries around the world. To assist in the brevity of writing this chapter, I am going to list in point form the disadvantages of red meat with a brief explanation, if needed.

Some Disadvantages of Eating Red Meat

1. No fiber.

2. No carbohydrates.

3. Too much protein.

4. Too much fat.

5. Loaded with cholesterol.

6. Vitamin content spotty.

7. Flesh harbors deadly bacteria. Since flesh is an

excellent insulator, not all microbes are killed by cooking.

8. Flesh is a disease-conveying agent (a long-recognized fact by the World Health Organization).

9. Flesh foods contain the highest concentra-tions of environmental poisons.

10. It does not supply fuel or energy in the same ready-to-use forms as carbohydrates.

11. Animals in many countries are raised on large quantities of antibiotics, hormones, and other drugs, and we are the ultimate recipients of these substances.

12. Flesh foods cause stress to the immune system. (After eating meat, the white blood cell count goes up, an indicator that the body recognizes toxins.)

13. The waste-containing blood stops moving in the animal's body at the time of death. The pink liquid you see on your plate after you have eaten roast beef contains the cow's red blood cells and other breakdown products of the cow's blood.

14. Meat has little fiber in it, thereby causing constipation. Due to the increased pressure with which the colon must squeeze the hard, fiberless fecal material, an unending flow of bacterial invaders are released into the bloodstream.

15. Ammonia is a byproduct of a high-flesh diet. Ammonia is toxic to the system.

16. The wastes and byproducts of meat overtax the kidneys. In meat eaters, the kidney has to work three times as hard to eliminate poisonous nitrogenous wastes.

17. Flesh is full of parasites. After the *E coli* scare

in 1993, the USDA advised the public to cook meat longer. This may kill more bacteria, but it also produces more carcinogens.

Note: *E coli* comes from the intestinal tracks of animals. It's your basic fecal matter.

18. During slaughter, it is almost impossible not to contaminate the meat with fecal and urine matter, due to the spillage of intestinal contents during the gutting of an animal carcass. Slaughterhouse workers say it is not uncommon for the contents of an animal's urine sac or diseased areas full of pus to spray all over the carcass.

19. You cannot cook out fecal matter.

20. The moment an animal dies, decomposition begins. In actual fact, the flesh begins rotting and starts to smell and discolor. Since gray-green

flesh is not aesthetically pleasing and does not sell well, thus begins the further injection of drugs, chemicals, and coloring agents to preserve the "red" appearance of meat.

21. The use of growth-promoting hormones is still legal in many countries.

22. Meat becomes very putrid after the long, arduous trip through the human intestine, which is not designed to handle animal flesh.

23. Putrefaction is accelerated in the heat of the body.

24. When the carcass is washed in the slaughterhouse, high-powered water is used, which further imbeds the bacteria into the flesh.

25. When the animal is killed, proteins in

the body coagulate and substances called ptomaines are formed. They result from the rapid decomposition and putrefaction of animal flesh.

26. The inspection process is spotty, at best. Animals go by very quickly, and to stop the processing line costs approximately $400 a minute. Few inspectors can withstand this pressure. Besides, it is almost impossible to inspect for parasites, as most are invisible to the eyes.

27. We eat flesh permeated with the violent energy of the pain and terror experienced at the time of slaughter. This is subtle, but it's probably one of the most under-researched aspects of what ultimately happens to us when eating an animal.

28. If you are a meat eater, you are contributing to the destruction of the ecology. The price tag on your piece of meat in the supermarket does

not include the loss of topsoil, air pollution, and water consumption.

29. No other item is as thoroughly tampered with as the meat people eat. This includes everything from reproduction (artificial insemination) to growth hormones to tranquilizers to feeding (antibiotics and insecticides). Manipulation takes places during every phase of the animal's life.

30. Four thousand people die each year as a result of meat getting caught in their throats (Dr. John McDougall). The number one product responsible for fatal choking in children is hot dogs.

5.6   The Hamburger and Hot Dog

Because of the growth of the hamburger and hot dog industry, a special section has been included on these products. The power of advertising and what it does to us is truly amazing. For instance, if we were to see a mangled human body on the side of the road, our stomachs would be upset. Yet we can put a mangled cow body in between two slices of bread, call it a hamburger, and our mouths water. If you ever saw a hamburger or hot dog being made from start to finish, only the most hardened of individuals would allow it to their lips. What makes the hamburger and hot dog such a risk is that bits and pieces of many cows go into it. Anything goes into it—the list includes guts and their secretions, organs, entrails, blood clots, toenails, scraps, intestinal matter, and abscesses, plus generous helpings of antibiotics and insecticides.

The hamburger, which is also called "the coronary bypass special" or "the indigestion burger," is actually a travesty to our society. Fast-food chains are proud when the number of hamburgers sold increases daily, but at whose expense? The majority of ground beef sold at hamburger outlets is actually ground-up dairy cows, whose flesh is not appealing enough to sell as whole steaks in the butcher section. The personal and environmental debt of a meat economy makes the U.S. national debt look minuscule.

It takes a long time for the consequences of meat eating to catch up with you—but when it does, it is traumatic. How many young children have lost their fathers due to a heart attack or cancer, simply because he could not control his craving for meat? Ironically, the very animals being killed for us to eat end up killing us. Meat is a graveyard food. The meat industry is very worried that more and more people will learn about the diseases caused by eating meat, about the rain forests and precious land being eroded and about the horrific conditions of factory farms. Dr. Neal Barnard, President of the Physician's Committee for Responsible Medicine, concludes, "The beef industry has contributed to more American deaths than all the wars of this century, all natural disasters, and all automobile accidents combined."

5.7 Chicken

In the last twenty years, many people have abandoned their dependence on red meat and have switched to chicken. They think they are doing themselves a favor by eating a supposedly healthier food. But chicken is not health food. Chickens are high in cholesterol, bacterial contaminates, and chemicals. Chicken is a pro-tein-dense food that contains the accumulated herbicides, pesticides, antibiotics, and hormones fed to the chicken during its factory farm production. A muscle is a muscle, whether it's a cow's, a fish's, or a chicken's. And the leaner the meat, the higher the cholesterol concentration. Calorie for calorie, chicken meat has more cholesterol than beef. Unfortunately, when people have high cholesterol, they are advised to eat chicken and fish. And when it doesn't go down, they are put on drugs. If the vast majority of the population were to eliminate animal products from their diet, cholesterol levels would go down dramatically within weeks.

In Chapter 2, I talked about factory farms. Now, let's take a look at what a typical chicken factory farm is like. The chickens are divided into broilers (those bred for flesh) and layers (those bred for laying eggs). Both live horrible lives. At birth, many males are discarded, while still alive, into trash cans to suffocate. Those chosen to live do so in filthy, litter-filled, crowded conditions. And if they had lived in the world naturally, their life spans would have been twelve to fifteen years. Here, in the factory farm, it is a scant four to five weeks. What is important to note is these chickens would not be ready to eat until about year or a year and a half if allowed a normal life, yet here they are fully grown at four to five weeks. How does this happen? Yes, more genetic manipulation for the sake of profits and the addition of growth-promoting hormones, which are ultimately consumed by humans.

The female, because she can lay eggs, gets a different life. She is cramped into a cage to live her entire life in an area the size of a piece of typing paper. Although her wingspan is an average of thirty-two inches, her cage is only eighteen inches wide. In these crowded conditions, the birds go berserk and peck at each other. Solution! Cut off their beaks with a hot blade—a very painful process. And some poor hack jobs result in major beak loss, leaving them unable to eat.

Chickens won't eat in the dark, so lights are kept on up to twenty-three and a half hours a day. Fluorescent light bulbs provide artificial light to stimulate laying. Therefore, they eat more and ultimately lay more eggs. Hens in the wild lay ten to twelve eggs a year. Battery hens lay around three hundred eggs a year. After twelve to fifteen months of faithfully laying eggs, she is cruelly transported and crudely slaughtered to end up in a soup tin or a can of dog food.

With Americans today consuming about twice as much chicken than they did in 1965, there is great demand for these creatures. The conditions in the slaughterhouse are so bad that before anyone thinks about eating chicken again, they should visit one. Speed is an important culprit in the contamination process. Eighty to ninety birds are processed per minute—a speed so quick that it turns things into a blur for the inspectors, who stare at carcasses eight hours a day. Current procedures make thorough inspection impossible.

Before they can be inspected, though, the birds have to be dismembered. This begins with the bird being strung upside down, its throat slit, and then shuttled off to a bath having a temperature of 140 degrees. When any creature dies, there is involuntary defecation; thus, we have instant sewage, or fecal soup. This cross-contamination is what allows bacteria to multiply. The scalding tank loosens feathers. The feathers are removed by a high-speed eviscerating machine, and bacteria are beaten into the skin. Frequently, the chickens' intestines are ruptured by the mechanical hands and bacteria-laden feces are spilled into the carcass.

It is easy to see why these birds are shipped out with problems ahead. The *Atlanta Constitution*

Journal newspaper interviewed eighty-four inspectors for an article which appeared on May 26, 1991. USDA inspector Ronnie Sarratt pointed out, "Thousands of diseased birds are shipped to stores every day. With yellow pus oozing from the birds, the workers are told to save them." The *Atlanta Constitution Journal* mentioned in the same article, "Each week throughout the South, millions of chickens, leaking yellow pus, stained with green feces, and contaminated by harmful bacteria or marred by lung and heart infections, cancerous tumors, or skin conditions, are shipped to customers."

By the time the birds leave the processing plant, chances are they have been infected with salmonella or campylobacter. Salmonella is a general term for about 2,000 closely-related types of bacteria. There are approximately 2.5 million cases of salmonella in the U.S. each year. Government studies have found about sixty-six percent of the chickens are contaminated with salmonella, and the bacteria that cause major problems are microscopic. Salmonella bacteria within a chicken breast grow quickly. They go from two to two million organisms in just two days.

Leukosis (chicken cancer) is also a problem. Dr. Virginia Livingston Wheeler says, "I consider the potential of cancer in chickens to be one hundred percent." Up until now, so much emphasis in cancer research has been focused on red meat. The chicken's turn is coming, and the results should be similar to those of red meat. Additionally, some chickens receive drugs such as Gentian Violet and Nitrofurons, which advance their growth and prevent disease, but are cancer-promoting in humans.

Since this stressful environment leaves the birds susceptible to infection and other diseases, they are given more antibiotics, the residues of which remain in the meat. For many centuries, chickens were not eaten because they are scavengers. On the farms, they were used to keep the land clean. And although they are smart, lovable, sentient beings, they were not considered clean. Interestingly, today's citizens, through clever advertising, have come to believe that eating two of the principal scavengers— chicken and fish—is part of a healthy lifestyle.

5.8 Fish

Contrary to what we think, the purpose of fish is to keep our rivers, lakes, and oceans clean. As scavengers, they have a remarkable ability to pick up whatever is thrown into the water. And in the last few decades, humans have poured mega-amounts of pollutants and toxins into their environment. The industrial waste and toxic chemicals that have spoiled so many waterways now pose a serious threat to anyone who eats fish. Thousands fall victim to illnesses caused by the consumption of contaminated fish. The new definition of fish could be: a blend of protein and fat seasoned with an array of toxic chemicals. In addition, the parasitic roundworms found in many fish can be translucent and hard to detect.

Fish occupy a high position on the food chain. Therefore, they are heavily contaminated. Toxins in the fish that humans eat are the result of biological magnification through "bioaccummulation" of fat-soluble substances in the oily muscles of fish. And the reason for this? The simplest forms of marine life engulf chemicals. These tiny creatures are ingested by small fish who are then eaten by larger fish, which humans ultimately consume. The Center for Disease Control says seafood is twenty-five times more likely to cause illnesses due to these chemicals (*Time* magazine, September 18, 1989). Unfortunately, the chemicals will be around for a long time. For example, PCB, which was banned in 1974, still shows up in concentration in fish today. Richard Gossett, of the Southern California Coastal Water Research Program, points out that fish eaters have five times more DDT in their blood than people who do not consume fish regularly.

Fish is not brain food, a myth that is still popular. In fact, it is the opposite. Methyl mercury, found in all ocean fish, is among the most toxic, naturally occurring substances on Earth. Mercury is a neuro-toxin, and it damages the brain and nervous system. With most of our fresh waters filled with excessive levels of lead, mercury, and toxic chemicals, fish is a wise product to avoid. It is almost impossible to tell if the fish is toxic. The toxins are odorless, tasteless, colorless, and indestructible. And even though there is a move to finally have fish inspected, it doesn't do much good.

Modern fishing methods also result in further contamination as we continue to rape our waters. Because the supply of fish closer to shore is sparse, fishermen must go further and further out, averaging four to twenty days on the water. The fish stored in the hold of the fishing boat, piled on top of one another, force the intestinal materials out of those at the bottom of the heap. Soon, all the fish in the hold are sloshing in a watery soup, thick with intestinal, fecal bacteria. These intestinal microbes hasten the spoilage of the fish, and the extra time spent on the boat allows an even greater growth of bacteria. Therefore, chemical preservatives, including antibiotics, are sprayed on the fish while they are in the boat's hold to retard decomposition until delivery to the fish market.

A subtle aspect of this trauma is that fish can and do survive for a long time (up to one hour) out of the water. During this suffocation, they are in great anxiety, and their tissue becomes flooded with their body's fear chemicals. Many religions do not permit the eating of fish, because they believe that subtle vibrations in the fish ultimately affect our consciousness.

Fish decompose faster than any other animal. If you have ever left a fish out in the sun on a hot summer day of about eighty degrees and returned three to four hours later, the stench is obvious. Can you imagine what is happening inside your body, as the fish traverses your intestinal system, which is 98.6 degrees?

Because fish is a high-protein food, precious calcium pours out of your body (see section on protein) each time you eat a piece of fish. Fish is devoid of carbohydrates and fiber, two items critical to optimal health. Freezing fish does not always help. Fish are cold-blooded creatures that live in cold environments. Many kinds of bacteria thrive in colder temperatures and are very comfortable in your refrigerator, multiplying easily there.

In addition to fish not being a healthy food, let's consider the ethics and environmental impact of fishing. Many people today are "fishtarians" (vegetarians who eat fish). They are hanging on to their last vestige of flesh. Many would like to go all the way and become full vegetarians, but they are addicted. Over the years, I have found the best approach to help them is by asking if they "support the concept of cheating." Since they inevitably answer no, I ask them how they can support an industry which exists on cheating. How do we catch fish? We cheat them. We use thin filament nets that snare them as they peacefully swim through the water; we use worms or lures with hidden hooks, etc.

When I was younger, I loved fishing. I quit fishing in 1970, but found myself fifteen years later in a hardware store in Parry Sound, Ontario, Canada, where some fishermen were testing new fishing rods. I had a flashback to how much fun it had been. But fun for whom? I quickly returned to reality. It's amazing to me now that in those days I had chosen to unwind and relax by stressing, mutilating, and killing other creatures. I am sorry.

And what about modern commercial fishing, with its long drift nets up to thirty miles in length? These walls of death are strip-mining the oceans as they take everything in their paths. The net sweeps an area the size of Ohio every night. In the North Pacific alone, over 1,000 miles of non-biodegradable nets are lost each year. They ghost fish for a long time. Not only is the industry over-fishing and disrupting the ecological balance of our oceans, but with long trips at sea, it is extremely energy intensive. And after all of these efforts, about fifty percent of the fish are fed to animals whose natural inclination is not to eat fish.

Perhaps one of the greatest travesties of the fishing industry is the large number of dolphins killed, particularly in the search for tuna. And even though "dolphin safe" is printed on the label, it is just a clever marketing ploy, as thousands of dolphins die each year during the catch. It is impossible to avoid catching dolphins. A permit from the Department of Commerce General allows for the legal slaughter of 20,500 dolphins in the U.S. How is it possible for us to support an industry that can take the life of a creature such as the dolphin, who has never harmed any human? Ironically, it is the dolphin who has saved many human lives. The next time you think about picking up a can of tuna or buying a tuna fish salad, picture those beautiful creatures with their wonderful smiles, frolicking in the water and then drowning in tuna nets.

5.9 Eggs

In the section on chickens you can see why eggs are sometimes referred to as "the breakfast of cruelty." Today's laying hen is a genetically manipulated freak. As we try to alter nature, the end product is usually not that good for us anyway. However, apart from the fact that modern egg production is accomplished through a stressful endeavor, the egg itself is not a food that works in harmony with your body.

First of all, it is an excellent source of artery-clogging cholesterol. One egg yolk contains approximately 220–260 mg. of cholesterol. Your body can only excrete about 100–300 mg. of cholesterol per day, so even an egg a day can be a detriment, as the cholesterol from an egg a day can cause the artery-clogging material to begin accumulating in the body. Many eggs are eaten invisibly, as a large number of processed foods, cakes, and cookies include eggs. So even if you don't eat eggs, if you fail to read food labels, you could be eating the equivalent of two to three eggs per day.

Eggs, like most chicken and fish, are high in protein and fat. The egg yolk is one of the densest concentrations of animal fat on the planet. It is made to fuel a baby chicken for twenty-one days.

Eggs decompose rapidly. If eggs are left unrefrigerated for more than a couple of hours, bacteria can multiply to dangerous levels, resulting in food poisoning. We should be suspect of any food that needs to be refrigerated, refrigeration being a recent invention.

Eating an egg is like eating glue. The fat of the egg yolk coats the red blood cells, making them stickier. In fact, in many societies the egg was, and still is, used as a glue for mending broken pots.

Eggs also contain an excess amount of sulfur. If you have ever smelled an egg which was broken open and left to rot, it is the sulfur that stinks. Sulfur is very hard on your liver and kidneys.

5.10   Dairy Products

This section of the book was the most difficult for me to write, as it is the only part where I am not comfortable. In short, the moral side of my consciousness abhors what the modern dairy industry has become in the last few decades; on the other hand, after many years of studying food choices and their effects on societies worldwide, I understand milk to be an integral part of all spiritual and religious traditions.

In fact, the oldest written scriptures, the *Vedas,* communicate the importance of milk for supplying nutrients to the finer tissues of the brain. ("Milk maintains the finer tissues of the brain for understanding the higher aims of life." *Srimad-Bhagavatam,* Canto 1, Chapter 8, Text 5) Great sages experienced that milk allows us to contemplate spiritual ideas. In ancient India, the Brahmans (saintly people) would often exist only on milk. They believed milk to be not only nutritious, but also essential for developing the brain cells necessary for spiritual understanding. Hence, my moral and ethical side is at odds with my spiritual and intellectual side. I will now present both sides and let you decide.

Raw milk is originally a pure food substance that is very helpful. It must be raw and fresh to have its full nutritive value. Milk, as we know it today, is far removed from the cow milk that is in a raw, natural, and non-manipulated state.

Milk was never meant to be drunk cold. Cold milk produces mucus. Even though a milkshake may taste wonderful, you have probably noticed the mucus in your throat afterward. Mucus is the body's way of counteracting the potentially damaging products introduced into the body. Hot milk helps calm nerves. Warm milk contains calcium and tryptophan, both of which help you sleep. This is why many societies drank (and still drink) warm milk before going to bed.

According to the original medical practice (Ayurvedic medicine), warm milk straight from the cow stimulates digestion, but cold milk causes arthritis, rheumatism, and toxic gases. In ancient times, when the cow was treated with love and respect, dairy products were pure food. The cow was revered—and still can be—as the surrogate mother of the human race. It was not uncommon for mothers to die at childbirth, and the cow was the only animal that could keep the child alive and in optimal health. Yet how do we treat such a valuable member of society in today's money-driven world? She is impersonally treated as an industrial product—from birth to slaughter. She is seen as financial stock and an object to be exploited. She is a product of the dairy industry.

Today's milk, like much of today's food, is dramatically altered. The alteration begins with artificial impregnation, which is nothing less than a violent rape conducted by men with sexual tools. In order to continue a supply of milk, the cow must be impregnated every year. Then the newborn calf is taken from the mother after only three days. This puts the mother in great distress. Following the separation, she cries most of the night; during the day, she searches for her calf. Instead of experiencing a loving, mother-child relationship, she is thrust into the role of an intensive milk producer. Sophisticated vacuum

121

milking machines suck her dry two to three times a day. She is forced to produce 15,000 pounds of milk per year (ten times what she would produce naturally). Some top-producing cows are forced to give up to 50,000 pounds of milk per year. As soon as her output slips, she is sold for slaughter. What normally would be a life span of twenty to twenty-five years is cut to three to five years. Her patient few years of serving count for nothing.

Left naturally, when a cow is done calving she will continue peacefully producing milk. A cow naturally produces more than its calf needs, which is only about one thenth of the milk in the udder. If she isn't milked, she will suffer great pain and eventually die. The cow is dependent upon humans. The cow is among the most placid of animals. She is patient, gentle, giving, and trusting. Yet, how do we treat her?

In the U.S. today, ninety-eight percent of our milk comes from factory farms. The demand for milk keeps the cows in constant stress, and they are, therefore, susceptible to disease. Then it is time for penicillin, antibiotics, and other drugs to stem the disease. Couple this with hormones for growth and production, along with environmental toxins, and you have polluted cow's milk.

However, pasteurization is seen as the savior. The milk is heated to between 161–170 degrees Fahrenheit. Not only does this destroy valuable enzymes, good bacteria, and nutrients, but it fuses the molecular structure of the protein content of milk, making it harder to digest.

A vegetarian who eats dairy products but no eggs is called a lacto-vegetarian. This is the category into which the highest number of vegetarians fall. In addition to milk, this includes butter, cheeses, and yogurt. One of the biggest concerns with butter is that it is one hundred percent fat and, therefore, raises your cholesterol. It is interesting to note that ghee (clarified butter, made by burning off the impurities in butter) does not raise cholesterol.

Yogurt is milk curdled by two strains of bacteria. It does not have as much lactose as milk. Therefore, it is easier to digest, as it contains bacteria which are beneficial to those who are lactose-intolerant. And it is well known for its ability to restore intestinal flora after a digestive upset. Only dairy products carry significant amounts of *lactobacillus acidophilus* (your friendly bacteria).

And if you are going to eat cheese, make certain it does not contain rennet. Rennet is a substance extracted from the stomach of a newborn calf and used in processing many commercial cheeses. There are soy-based cheeses, most of which at this time contain a trace of casein so the cheese will stretch when melted. Most of these "health food" cheeses are made with vegetable-derived rennet.

In closing, I would be remiss if I did not discuss the veal industry, since veal is a byproduct of the dairy industry. This is the ultimate in cruelty. As mentioned, newborn male calves are taken from their mothers one to three days after birth and live their brief lives confined to wooden stalls just large enough to hold them. These innocents are chained at the neck and unable to move for the duration of their lives. They are fed an antibiotic-laced liquid diet of a milk substitute that is deliberately iron deficient, helping to create the pale, white meat of veal. Sixteen weeks later, these young creatures are bound for the slaughterhouse and, ultimately, to a plate as Veal Parmesan.

5.11   Grains

For most of the world's population, grains are still the staple of their diet. Rice is the staff of life for fifty percent of the world's population and was originally the most cultivated grain in the world. Now, it is wheat. This is principally due to the growing of so much wheat for animal feed. Grains are experiencing a revival. No longer perceived as food for the poor, rice, wheat, barley, etc. are on the increase among the better informed. Grains (unrefined) are full of valuable fiber, are cholesterol-free, and contain a minimum amount fat.

All ethnic menus have either grains and/or beans as the foundation of their meals—Italians and pasta, Chinese and rice, Mexicans and beans, etc. The wisest move you can make to benefit the quality of your life is to do likewise.

5.12   Legumes (Beans, Peas, etc.)

Legumes, like grains, are a first-class food. They are wholesome, filling, and inexpensive. A legume is anything which grows in a pod. Legumes can be stored for a long time without much loss of the valuable nutri-ents they provide. Beans are a perfect food and a nutritional powerhouse. They are complex carbohydrates, full of vitamins and minerals with almost no sodium.

Apart from being perceived as low-class food, beans have a mild drawback in that they cause gas. This is due to the fact that two of the carbohydrates contained in beans are not completely digested in the stomach. As these undigested carbohydrates travel through our system, the intestinal tract has a feast digesting them and, thus, releasing gas. The gas is not dangerous, just embarrassing and possibly uncomfortable.

You can, however, de-gas beans to a certain extent by soaking the beans in water, frequently changing the water, bringing them to a boil for three to five minutes, and then setting them aside to soak in water four to six hours before cooking in a fresh pot of water. Also, there is a new product called "Beano" that does a good job of de-gassing legumes. (It is the missing enzyme in liquid form.)

Supposedly, a few drops on the first bite is all you need.

As Dr. Michael Klaper, one of America's leading doctors on nutrition, points out, "It is interesting to note that the more frequently beans and legumes appear in the diet, the less gas there is, as the bacterial population changes to less gas-producing species."

The soybean is revered in many cultures for its versatility. For many, tofu is a relatively new part of their food choices. It is the Eastern counterpart of cheese; it comes from cooking and then pureeing soybeans into curd. It is a culinary chameleon, having the ability to absorb the flavors of many ingredients.

5.13 Vegetables

Unfortunately, the first six letters of vegetarian and vegetable are the same. This results in many people thinking that vegetarians eat only vegetables. Although vegetables are one of the key ingredients of a vegetarian diet, there are many more classes of plant foods. The "staff of life," the basis of diet historically and internationally, is grain. Wheat produces cereals, farina, and flour. And there is rice, corn, and millet. Trees produce fruits and nuts in great variety. And from grass and flowers come the gifts of living creatures—milk and honey.

Consider all the spices and flavors of ethnic cuisines (Italian, Oriental, Thai, Indian, Mexican, etc.) with all their wonderful soups, sandwiches, casseroles, pasta dishes, and desserts. Plant foods are modest in calories, have zero cholesterol, and are extremely nutrient-dense. They are rich in nutrients vital to warding off environmental toxins and preventing disease. These include vitamins C, E, and beta-carotene—all powerful antioxidants found almost exclusively in plants.

All essential nutritive materials are formed in the plant kingdom to be cultivated in gardens, humankind's original work place.

5.14   Fruits

Fruits are essential to our well-being. They should provide the bulk of our natural sugar intake. However, with the advent of processed food full of fat and processed sugar, people have left fruits aside—so much so that a large number of people in the U.S. are not getting enough fruit each day.

Fruit sugars are converted from starch to sugar while ripening under the influence of the sun. Fruits are your quickest source of energy and are an excellent food for breakfast. They require very little energy to digest (they go through your stomach in twenty to thirty minutes), and for this reason should, ideally, be eaten alone.

Additionally, they are cholesterol-free and fat-free, as well as high in fiber, carbohydrates, and water. Although there are about three thousand identified fruits worldwide, only about one hundred are imported into the U.S.

If you like fruit juices, buy a juicer and make it yourself. Most of the commercial juices are very diluted and have many additives. If you make your own juices, drink them right away while the vitamins and minerals are most potent. If you store it, put a little olive oil on top to form an air-tight film. Fruits are a wonderful gift of nature and should be an integral part of your optimal food choices.

5.15   Fiber

In the Western world, a flesh-based diet, which is deficient of fiber, has resulted in chronic constipation for many people. Fiber is that portion of plant food that the human digestive enzymes cannot break down. Manufacturers remove it because they think it has no value. Until recently, fiber has been a largely neglected component of food, mainly because it has no nutritional value. Fiber itself does not provide calories, since it is not absorbed or digested by the body. Its purpose has been misunderstood. However, the health advantages of a high-fiber diet are clear.

Fiber resists digestion and absorption and, therefore, moves matter more rapidly through the colon. In addition, fiber tends to attract and bond with fat. It also absorbs water to help keep the contents of the stool soft. Without water, the contents compact and we become constipated. Fiber thus facilitates regular bowel movements. A shorter transit time minimizes the bowel wall's contact with carcinogens. Dietary fiber binds and inactivates carcinogens that lead to cancer and heart disease-causing cholesterol. Overall, fiber keeps your bowels clean and healthy. The insoluble fiber, which will not mix with water, is the "Drano" of the digestive tract. An added bonus of high-fiber foods is that they tend to make you feel full. And because you stop eating sooner, fewer calories are consumed.

As mentioned, flesh foods are completely lacking in fiber, but fiber is found in abundance in fruits, vegetables, and in wholesome, unprocessed grains. Complex carbohydrates have a superior fiber content. Whole foods contain much more fiber than juices. Raw fruits and vegetables act as nature's broom. The cellular fibers act as tiny brooms or scrub brushes.

There is one myth surrounding fiber: that it will inhibit the absorption of iron and other vital minerals. This myth was laid to rest when Dr. Colin Campbell, then Chairman of the Department of Nutritional Biochemistry at Cornell University, did his now famous Cornell-China-Oxford study. The Chinese have a very high-fiber intake (an average of thirty-four grams per day per person compared to the U.S. average of ten grams per day), yet they have high levels of iron in their blood.

Americans used to average forty-five grams of fiber per day, until we became dependent upon fiber-free foods (meat, chicken, fish, and eggs) as our staples. One industry that has thrived due to the resulting abundance of constipation has been the laxative industry. If we were to put fiber back into our diets, you had better sell the stocks you hold in companies depending on the sale of laxatives for their survival.

5.16 Vitamins

Fresh fruits and vegetables are truly the richest sources of vitamins and minerals. Ideally, these nutrients should come from gardens and orchards, not pharmaceutical labs. Most people in modern society depend on the shelves in pharmacies as their main source of vitamins. No one could afford to extract vitamins from food for commercial sale. Yet, billions of dollars are spent each year on manufactured vitamins. Unfortunately, within hours of the consumption of these vitamins, most are found en route to the local sewage treatment plant.

With the advent of the current popularity of vitamins, many studies were conducted to see if it was necessary to take supplemental vitamins. The conclusion was, generally, no—until recently, with the discovery that extra vitamins can potentially be very helpful in fighting cancer and heart diseases. Today, our food, air, water, soil—even our homes and offices—are infused with radiation, drugs, and chemical pollutants. As a result, our immune and detoxification systems are weakened to varying degrees, so supplemental vitamins may be necessary for many people.

Contrary to popular belief, vitamins do not provide energy. Their principal role is that of an activator, promoting chemical reactions in your body. However, they are used up in these reactions; and since they cannot be made by the body, we must consume additional vitamins. They are needed in minute quantities, so a large intake is not advisable. Balance is very important. Too much of a nutrient can be as damaging as too little. Since some vitamins are excreted slowly, they can build up to toxic levels. (Vitamin A, for example, produces toxic symptoms when taken in excess. Vitamin C, though, can be consumed in massive amounts for certain therapies.)

There are two kinds of vitamins: water soluble and fat soluble. Water soluble vitamins are easily destroyed by heating. For example, because

Vitamin C is very fragile, when you cook fruit (an excellent source of Vitamin C), you destroy most of the Vitamin C. Fat soluble vitamins, on the other hand, are fairly stable.

How much of each vitamin should we have? Even the committee that sets the RDAs (the Required Daily Amounts) doesn't recommend definitive dosage amounts for optimal health. However, there are some guidelines, and it is advisable for you to have periodic blood tests to see if you are deficient in any vitamin or mineral.

Special note should be made here about Vitamin B12. This vitamin plays an important role in assisting the proper formation of the body's nerves and red blood cells. The biggest concern for Vitamin B12 deficiency is in vegans (vegetarians who do not consume any animal products, including dairy). Since B12 is produced exclusively by bacteria, animals are perceived as a better source because of bacterial growth in their intestines. This is why a lacto-vegetarian would not have a deficiency. However, you would get all the Vitamin B12 necessary by regularly eating vegetables from a well-manured soil. If we were taking our vegetables directly from the garden, we would be getting ample B12, as it is very plentiful in the surface layers of vegetables. However, our commercially prepared food is so thoroughly washed that B12 is almost non-existent. We are so sterile oriented that we also destroy friendly bacteria. At any one time, we have a three to eight-year supply of B12 in our bodies, yet there is concern for deficiencies. Dr. John McDougall, author of many books on nutrition, points out that there are less than a dozen B12 deficiencies in the world, and most of these cases occur in meat eaters.

5.17 Minerals

Minerals are metals from Earth's crust. Plants extract minerals from the ground and deliver them to us through the fruits and vegetables they bear. A sensible diet provides all the minerals you need. Examples of minerals you are probably familiar with are calcium, sodium, potassium, phosphorous, and magnesium. The soil also provides us with trace minerals we need, such as zinc and copper.

Minerals are building blocks, and each one of them has specific functions. It is not helpful to have a surplus in your body. If we were to eat one mineral in excess, most of it would be blocked from absorption, as our body protects us from such dietary foolishness.

Special mention should be made of iron, as people are often concerned about getting enough. There is a misconception that iron from meat is better than iron from vegetables. It is true that the iron found in meat is easier to digest, but vegetarians get just as much iron because vegetables provide Vitamin C as well, which aids in the absorption of iron. Generally, vegetarians have few cases of iron deficiency anemia (*Vegetarian Times*, September 1991), largely because the body is very efficient in recycling iron.

5.18   Sugar

Sweet is one of our six basic tastes. In fact, sweetness is the only innate taste preference we have as infants. Unlike fat, sugar causes no life-threatening illnesses. There are no conclusive studies that show that any type of sugar causes hypoglycemia or diabetes. However, the excess amounts consumed by Western societies is ludicrous and dangerous, and can be an accomplice to foster other diseases. We have gone overboard. In 1790, the average intake of sugar per day was eight grams. Today, it is around 125 grams. Over one year (365 days) that is one hundred pounds of sugar.

When sugar enters the bloodstream, it is readily absorbable. The advantage of natural sugars from fruits is that they seep into the blood more slowly and evenly because they are eaten combined with fiber, which retards absorption. Refined sugar jolts the body, has no fiber, and is a non-nutritive substance. If it isn't needed right away, it is stored as fat. Alcohol and sweets are excellent flab generators.

Western society is exposed to highly sweetened foods from infancy. Most of our sugar is found in the processed foods we eat. For example, a twelve-ounce can of soda can contain ten teaspoons of sugar. We have a major dependency on sugar. It is this dependency that causes us to eat foods that fill us up but do not have any health benefits. Actually, if you focus on a more natural-based vegetarian diet, your intake of sugar will decrease automatically.

The majority of this chapter has focused on what not to eat. Most of you know you should eat fruits and vegetables and that vitamins and minerals are important, but many of you may currently have foods in your diet which are not beneficial for your optimal health. Even a hundred years ago we were better off, as we had a more active lifestyle and a more healthful environment. But as pointed out in Chapter 2, our more affluent, modern society has brought with it numerous problems, which I will address in the next chapter.

Diseases of the Affluent

Disease doesn't just happen. It accumulates. Long before you are aware of any symptoms, there has been a long period of degeneration. Illness is a sign that our body has strayed from a state of equilibrium. There is an energy crisis in the body. Disease means lack of ease. Today we are very much oriented to curing the symptom and not the problem. If you have a headache, you take a pill. A pill may eliminate the pain, but it does nothing for the problem itself.

A majority of our current killer diseases are diet-related; we can control our destinies by controlling our tongues. The body has the intelligence to restore itself to health—if we give it a chance. But we are so addicted to certain foods and drinks that our poor bodies are in a constant state of turmoil. Couple this with external forces that are eroding our health, and it makes our chances of feeling great for any length of time a rare occurrence.

Various societies have their theories on why illness occurs. The Chinese believe that energy imbalance is the root of all illness. The Buddhists believe that it is because of stagnant foods (constipation). The Hindus believe that if the food is not offered, we receive bad karma from the killing of any living entity (plants included). What we do know for sure is that the closer a country's diet is to the Western model, the more their people suffer from the following diseases of the affluent.

6.1   Heart Attacks

When it comes to heart attacks, we largely control our destiny. Yet, every minute in the U.S., two people have heart attacks. One dies, and one lives. And people accept this as NORMAL. Heart disease has become a socially accepted epidemic. We are not supposed to be fifty years of age with our chests split open. Eighty percent of males in the U.S. die prematurely, and every year the number of heart attacks among teenagers increases. Women, due to their body design for preservation of the species, are generally protected up to menopause. However, the number of heart attacks begins to rise shortly after menopause, and they catch up with their male counterparts six to eight years following menopause.

Signs of a heart attack are a crushing, pressure-like pain in the chest behind the breastbone, though the symptoms may be as varied as pain in the jaw or a steady ache in the left arm or center of the back. Sensation may spread to the shoulders, neck, or arms. If it lasts for more than two minutes, you could be having a heart attack. Other signs are dizziness, sweating, and shortness of breath. If you think you've had a heart attack, go to your doctor. A heart attack occurs from the cutoff of oxygen-rich blood to some part of the heart. This is usually due to a blood clot, which gets stuck in an already narrowed artery. Lack of oxygen leads to the death of the heart muscle. The three, pencil-slim coronary arteries must stay open. There are no heart attacks without closed arteries.

The first symptom of a heart attack can be sudden death. This is due to the fact that arteries do not have any nerves to warn us of ongoing damage. You can't feel your arteries slowly being clogged with fat. Atherosclerosis progresses until a blood clot forms on the surface of a cholesterol-laden plaque, sealing off blood flow to the vital heart muscle. Suddenly, a life ends. Most who survive a heart attack didn't even know they were at risk.

In 1992, there were 1.6 million heart attacks and 270,000 strokes in the U.S. A stroke is when a blocked artery prevents oxygen from getting to the brain. Fifty percent of the United States death toll is due to heart attacks and strokes.

The only way to lower heart disease risk is to lower your cholesterol level. Patients with narrowed arteries in the heart nearly always experience chest pains after eating a high-fat diet. Diet and heart disease are directly co-related, and the onset of war often verifies this. During hard times, people eat less flesh, and thus the number of heart attacks decreases. Never was this more evident than in Iraq in 1991 when sanctions were imposed. Heart attacks, which were the number

147

one cause of death, dropped dramatically (May 8, 1992, *Daily Independence*, Tokyo).

Despite the fact that seventy-five percent of the world's population never have heart attacks, coronary care units in the U.S. are overflowing. Coronary artery disease was a rarity in the early 1900s, yet, in 1992, 400,000 heart bypass operations were performed in the United States alone. It is now the most common major operation, and it's a big moneymaker as well. Yet, it doesn't solve the problem—it just prolongs it. After the bypass operation, if you don't change your diet and lifestyle, the arteries continue to close at the same or an accelerated rate (Dr. John McDougall).

Unless you change your eating habits (and cease smoking, regularly exercise, and reduce stress), a bypass operation is avoiding the real problem. As pointed out, one out of every two people who have heart attacks dies. If you are

148

one of those who has had a heart attack and are reading this, treat this warning as a telegram urging you to change the way you eat. Otherwise, you'll have another date with your cardiologist soon.

A recent study by the German Cancer Research Center in Hamburg found that the death rate from heart disease was fifty percent less in vegetarians than that of the general population.

6.2   High Blood Pressure

High blood pressure is referred to as "the silent killer." It is like a flashing red light, warning that you are at risk. In some cultures of the world, high blood pressure is unheard of, regardless of age. High blood pressure is very much diet-related, the result of living too luxuriously for too many years. When plaque builds up on the arterial walls, the heart must beat harder to get the blood through a more constricted space, which results in a higher blood pressure.

How is high blood pressure treated? Almost always with drugs. Yet, within the first day of switching to a diet low in saturated fats, free of animal origin and salt, blood pressure begins to fall. Blood pressure is measured by two numbers (for example, 140/80). The top (first) number represents the squeezing phase of your heartbeat; the bottom number is the pressure when you are relaxed. Borderline hypertension is 140/90, so your goal should be around 110/70.

6.3   High Cholesterol

High cholesterol is a problem in the Western world, and as usual, averages bring misconceptions. Your doctor may tell you that your cholesterol count of 230 mg. is "average." But what you are not told is that 230 mg. is also average in coronary care units—so you had better get your will ready. To be truly safe, you need to get your count under 150 mg. Since roughly eighty million Americans have elevated cholesterol counts, this is a serious issue. High cholesterol is definitely linked to heart disease.

Diet is the cornerstone of all cholesterol therapy. Neither exercise nor the leaner meats lower cholesterol, as previously discussed. Cholesterol can be lowered about twenty-five percent in three to four weeks on a lacto-vegetarian diet (using minimal dairy products). To begin lowering cholesterol, stop eating someone else's cholesterol. Cholesterol is found in the liver of all animals. If it doesn't have a liver, it cannot produce cholesterol. Blood cholesterol levels can be the barometer of your life span, a crystal ball to your future health.

6.4   Atherosclerosis

Until recently, there was a theory that hardening of the arteries and clotting of the blood were companions of old age. We now know that atherosclerosis is largely influenced by lifestyle and is a direct result of too much cholesterol in the blood. The arteries deliver the blood; the veins return it. Veins do not develop atherosclerosis because they do not have a middle layer of muscle tissue, which is rich in protein and is needed to start plaque formation. Without protein, plaque formation cannot begin. The entire body is dependent upon an arterial system that should be flexible, elastic, and clean. A person is as old as their arteries. However, with today's Western-style diet, children begin the atherosclerotic buildup as early as six months of age, although a significant showing does not occur until around eleven years of age.

In 1990, Dr. Dean Ornish, in Berkeley, California, presented a landmark study showing that it is now possible to reverse atherosclerotic buildup by way of a vegetarian diet, exercise, and meditation. Dr. Ornish's program has had enormous success. Actually, in 1986, Dr. Blankenhorn and his associates at the University of Southern California also demonstrated that atherosclerotic buildup could be reversed by lowering blood cholesterol through an increased intake of the drug niacin.

6.5   Cancer

Cancer is the number one cause of death in the U.S. Every year, about one million people learn they have cancer (American Cancer Institute), and the high-fat, Western diet is the leading cause of cancer (Lancet, 140–162, 1992). The lifestyle of many people today is conducive to getting cancer because of poor diet, exposure to too many toxins, and a high level of stress.

Cancer is the abnormal growth of our cells. It begins with a single cell whose blueprint (DNA) has been corrupted. Growth is slow, doubling about every one hundred days. Normal cells live side by side in a neighborly manner, but cancer cells divide and grow uncontrollably with no regard for the cells around them. They push the normal cells aside to form a lump called a tumor. After about ten years, it is the size of an eraser. By the time it is visible, the cancer cells have almost always spread throughout the body. Sir MacFarlane Burnett, the British scientist and Nobel Prize winner for his work in immunology, found that 100,000 cells can become cancerous in the body each day. But if the immune system is strong and functioning normally, it will immediately destroy these cells. He found that tumors will disappear.

Cancer is not genetic. Do not blame your parents. It is a disease of bad habit. The Western diet is a recipe for cancer. Carcinogens are formed when fish or flesh is charred or burned. This burning creates a kind of chemical element called methylcholanthrene, which is a powerful carcinogen. Additionally, all fats are involved in the growth of certain kinds of cancer cells (Dr. John McDougall).

In the last fifty years, the overall death rate attributed to cancer has not been significantly reduced, despite the billions of dollars spent on research. In fact, so many people are trying to find a cure for cancer that it is predicted if a cure were ever found, an estimated 1.5 million people would be out of jobs in the U.S. alone.

Lots of research and resulting evidence point to a vegetarian diet as a major positive step in both preventing and curing cancer naturally. The Heidelberg German Cancer Research

Center found that vegetarians are twice as resistant to tumor cells. Dr. Colin Campbell says, "If we switch from animal to plant protein, we basically turn off the further growth of tumors." In a landmark study of 129 cancer patients who had received the best medical care, the group receiving nutritional support lived twelve times longer than those who did not (Hoffer, A., Pauling, L., *Orthomolecular Medicine,* 1990). A theory that is gaining tremendous popularity in cancer cure is to not feed the cancer patient any protein for two months; the body will feed on the cancer cells for its protein.

Unfortunately, today's medical establishment has a high propensity toward chemotherapy, even though these procedures seldom extend lives and they cause serious toxic side effects. These treatments are invasive (just as is open-heart surgery) and, once again, only treat symptoms. It is unfortunate, since there are so many alternative, nonpoisonous treatments available.

If you have been diagnosed with cancer, the most important step you can take is to choose a diet that will build up your immune system while starving the cancer cells. Since cancer develops at some time in all bodies, we should do something to protect ourselves.

6.6   Obesity

The majority of populations in every developed nation of the Western world is overweight. And what is alarming is that childhood obesity in the U.S. has reached epidemic proportions. Children have twenty percent more body fat than their counterparts in the 1970s, and this is not limited to the U.S. I'm amazed when I visit countries such as Japan, Singapore, and Hong Kong and see what the introduction of a Western-style diet has done to them—lots of fat kids. The fact that America's kids watch television six to seven hours per day and mandatory physical education has been eliminated in almost every state has played a major role. Couple this with an early dependence on fat-filled foods, and the children have a much shorter life ahead of them. And women in the Western world have often looked upon pregnancy as a license to eat; thus their mucus-filled, overweight newborns laboriously and painfully enter a world waiting to stuff them to an early death.

All obesity is risky. It is not genetic. Eighty to eighty-five percent of fat people have some disease which is related to their obesity. You gain weight by eating too much and/or exercising too little. By definition, most experts consider obesity to be when a person is twenty percent or more above the appropriate weight for his or her height.

Extra weight taxes your body and its organs. For each pound of fat, an additional one mile of capillaries is required. And what about the "bag of cement" many men carry on top of their stomach? It's estimated that for each extra ten pounds in this area, the spinal disk must withstand an additional fifty to one hundred pounds of extra pressure. Over the long haul, the vertebrae grind together until they finally corrode and crumble.

And what about the economics of fat? Weight loss is a big business, particularly with women. Women always think of (or see) themselves as fatter or heavier than they actually are, while men see themselves as lighter or smaller than reality. In the U.S. alone, fifty percent of the women are actively dieting, and many of them are looking to purchase the "magic bullets" (pills, drinks, etc.) that will help the fat disappear. In addition, we have to make our spectator seats in theaters and sports arenas bigger every few decades. In the early 1950s, the average seat was 15–17 inches wide, whereas today it is 20–22 inches wide—and that still isn't big enough for far too many people. Larger individual seats mean less overall seats and, thus, higher ticket prices.

Obesity seems to be related more to what we eat than to how much. In China, the average person eats twenty percent more per body weight than Americans, yet obesity is rare. They just don't eat the volume of fat that Americans eat. The fat we eat becomes the fat we wear. Many overweight people actually eat less in volume than their thin friends. This is usually due to the fact that they are dieting and still aren't eating the right foods. Also, they have less energy to exercise. Weight control is much easier on a vegetarian diet than on any other. If you switch from a fat-based diet to a starch-based diet (breads, pastas, rice, vegetables, etc.), you will almost always lose weight effortlessly.

The body has unlimited capacity to store fat. And fat transforms into gained weight because it is stored in the body more easily than carbohydrates or proteins. Your body loves to convert dietary fat into body fat because the transformation takes a small amount of energy. Fat cells shrink or swell, depending upon the fat in them, but they never disappear. Women are particularly concerned about the cellulite on their thighs. It is no different than other fat in their body. Women have a thinner outer layer of skin and the fat cells are larger and more rounded. It is the straining against the irregular bands of tissue that gives the "cottage-cheese effect." Cellulite also responds (along with a low-fat vegetarian diet) to a therapeutic program of nightly sessions of twenty minutes of heat applied to the area, followed by vigorous fingertip massage to increase circulation and fat metabolism.

In earlier societies, fat people represented prosperity. Fat was a class symbol of higher status, because it meant one didn't work in the fields and had lots of food to eat. However, it has become less and less associated with opulence. Being overweight and overfat is dangerous to your health. I read a wonderful quote recently which is very appropriate: "The body you carry for the rest of your life is baggage. Any excess baggage shortens the trip."

6.7 Osteoporosis

Osteoporosis is a disease of excess. We have a dietary epidemic of osteoporosis throughout societies worldwide. The incidence of osteoporosis is most common in countries that consume the greatest number of animal products (U.S., England, Finland, Sweden, and Israel). It is almost non-existent in third world countries or tribal societies in which physical activity is the norm. Asians and Africans have the strongest teeth and bones, while women in the Western world are hemorrhaging calcium from their bones. The definition of osteoporosis is "porous bones" (osteo means bones; porous means hole). Although everybody loses a little bone with age, excess loss (osteoporosis) is a degenerative disease which is not normal. It is principally related to what we eat. Consumption of any kind of animal flesh will lead to more acidity in the body, as measured in the urine. To buffer the excess of amino acids, the body leaches calcium from the bones. In medical terms, this is called "protein-induced hypercalceria."

Osteoporosis kills lots of people. But we can prevent further loss by simply lowering the protein content of our diet. Each time you eat a piece of fish, chicken, or red meat, precious calcium pours out of your body. There is also evidence that, with a good exercise program, osteoporosis can be reversed. Osteoporosis can also be affected by other factors such as lack of exercise, caffeine ingestion, cigarette smoke, alcohol, refined sugars, high-salt diets, and, yes, some element of genetics.

6.8 Stress

Life today seems to be getting tougher, becoming faster and more demanding than ever. There are forces working on you every day, trying to disintegrate your body. Attendance at stress seminars is at an all-time high. Like the weather, everybody's talking about it.

If you ask most people today about it, they say they are more stressed than they were five years ago. Most say they don't use their free time to relax or have fun, but rather to recuperate from working. However, it's important to realize that stress has always been a part of life. Do you think that the pioneers, as they settled on new land, were stress-free, with responsibilities like searching for food and shelter? What we have today is just a different kind of stress, and we are not handling it well. Sales of anti-anxiety drugs are increasing every year. Part of the difficulty is that we are stressing our bodies internally by pouring the wrong foods and drinks into it. As we poison our bodies, our health is not at its peak. So, when external forces hit us (finances, work, marital problems, and disasters), we don't have appropriate energy to deal with them—and we turn to maladaptive practices (drugs, alcohol, smoking, etc.).

What we need to realize is that stress should be a performance enhancer—it should motivate us. But instead, it has become a scapegoat.

Instead of managing stress, we let it manage us. All stress can harm us by weakening or blunting our immune system. This is why it is essential to be in good health, as a fit body is always able to handle stress better.

The three best-known antidotes for handling stress are as follows:

1. Exercise. It burns up stress physiologically. People always feel better and more relaxed following a good workout.

2. Carve out some quiet time each day. Researchers agree that spending a small part of each day in a totally relaxed state is enormously therapeutic for one's mind and body.

3. Stop trying to be in control of everything. You are not in charge of everything. Events will happen. A positive attitude will always help you deal with whatever comes your way. Stress is a fact of life, just don't make it a way of life.

Hopefully, you now understand that a majority

of the diseases that are killing most of us are a result of what goes on our forks, chopsticks, or hands. Nutrition is the crown pillar of health, but its very important companion is what we are now going to look at . . .

Exercise

About eight years after officially leaving the professional tennis tour, I discovered that my size 32 tennis shorts no longer fit. I had been able to wear a size 32 since I was 17 years old. But now, at age 37, some 20 years later, I had to give in to a size 34. This was discouraging. And a check on the scale showed that I had gone from 150 pounds to 175 pounds.

How could this happen? I was still playing and teaching tennis six to eight hours per day. Granted, a 34-inch waist wasn't bad when compared to my friends, who had ballooned out further than that. Nevertheless, it was disturbing.

I vowed to lose it—and once I did, I would never wear anything larger than a 32-inch pair of shorts again.

But how was I going to accomplish this? I disliked running. I was a terrible swimmer. Bicycling was too dangerous on the crowded roads of Honolulu. Cross-country skiing? . . . not in Hawaii. And walking was for older people (my misconception in 1983). I knew it was going to have to be an aerobic activity, the only effective way to lose weight and keep it off. I knew that aerobics wasn't just a dance class, but I was reluctant to go because my dancing was worse than my swimming.

Fortunately, at this time a friend of mine, who was a rugby player and former athlete, was also twenty-five pounds overweight, and he also wanted to lose the extra weight. So we made a bet. A ridiculous sum would go to whoever lost the weight first. We signed up for an aerobics class at the local YMCA from 5:30–6:30 PM Monday through Friday and 9:00–10:00 AM Saturday mornings. We were committed, six days a week.

My friend, who was a lot more coordinated than I, stood in the middle of the group while I stood in the back. Five minutes into the first class, any misconception I had harbored about aerobics not being for athletes was dispelled. I thought my heart and lungs were going to fly out of my chest. I became an instant believer that there was something of value to this aerobics class.

Five and one-half weeks later, I had won the bet. But it wasn't until a number of years later that I understood the reason why I had shed twenty-five pounds so easily while my friend had lost only one pound, even though we had gone to the same workouts together. What I learned was what researchers had concluded: You cannot effectively lose weight from an aerobic movement program unless you alter your diet first. As well, without proper nutrition you may not have enough energy to exercise at a level you would like. I mentioned earlier that I had switched to a vegetarian diet, while my friend was still filling up on protein. Under normal circumstances, one should only lose two to three pounds per week, but I lost mine effortlessly. (Well, it was effortless after the first week of adjusting to the new program.)

Although a change in your food choices should come first, without exercise as a partner, it is unlikely you'll keep the weight off. But as you know, apart from the weight issue, exercise has an enormous number of benefits. The human body is built to exercise. Doing anything physical is much better than remaining inactive. After a good workout, you won't hear anyone say, "I wish

I hadn't done that." I have outlined the top twenty advantages of exercise, with a brief explanation for each.

Top Twenty Advantages of Exercise

1. Flushes Poisons Out of the Body.

During exercise, your body temperature rises several degrees. This helps kill bacteria. When you exercise, your body releases the same proteins it does when it is fighting bacteria, and it produces a higher number of white cells. Toxins are also released through perspiration. And, finally, during an aerobic workout, poisons are released through the mouth.

2. Stimulates Immune System.

Exercise helps muscles contract to push fluid through the one-way valves. Sitting down or inactivity slows circulation and stagnates the blood.

3. Reduces Amount of Fat in the Body.

Apart from the fact that excess fat is damaging to your health, fat stores many toxins. Exercise literally "turns on" your metabolism and liberates calories.

4. Strengthens Lungs and Heart.

Life is movement, and the heart craves exercise. When the heart is strong, it beats less often. Since there is no way to exercise the heart, lungs, and blood vessels directly, exercise places a demand on the cardiovascular system. Lack of exercise makes one two times more likely to develop coronary heart disease (Center for Disease Control).

5. Raises Basic Metabolic Rate.

This means you will burn more calories—not only during a workout, but also while at rest. The metabolic rate can remain elevated for up to twelve hours after exercise.

6. Increases Number of Red Blood Cells.

More red blood cells increases the carrying capacity of oxygen to the muscles. Therefore, you don't quit as soon.

7. More Oxygen to the Cells.

The purpose of exercise is to get oxygen to cells. If cells don't get oxygen, they die. The muscles of a physically fit person are better able to extract oxygen from circulating blood.

8. Stronger Bones.

Bones strengthen and thicken, just like muscles, when exercised or subjected to heavy loads or gravity. Tennis players always have bigger bones in the arm they play with. This is important to know, as there are still too many people who think they get stronger bones by pouring vast amounts of calcium into their body.

9. Builds Up Muscles.

There are approximately 630 muscles in the body, and if you don't use them, they atrophy.

The human body actually breaks down when it is not being used. So, the more you use your muscles, the better they get. A well-exercised bicep doesn't deteriorate; it gets stronger.

10. Peripheral Circulation Increased.

This is a big one, because alternate routes for blood are opened up in the event the main artery is blocked. This may save your life.

11. Keeps Joints More Mobile.

There is less degeneration of joints. Too many people rust out too soon.

12. Raises HDL (The Good Cholesterol).

HDL is believed to be an arterial cleanser.

13. Reduces Potential Cancer Risks.

Scientists believe that exercise reduces the risk of cancer by causing good activity in the colon, whereby food moves out of the body at a faster rate. In talking with doctors in the East, they all believed this to be one of the principal keys to good health.

14. Appetite Depressed After Exercise.

This usually occurs for one to two hours following the exercise. It limits the craving and desire to eat more.

15. Helps Store More Glycogen.

A fit person stores more glycogen in the muscle (between ten to fifty percent more than an unfit person) and, thus, gains a greater ability for endurance workouts.

16. Helps Overcome Weariness.

The best remedy for fatigue or weariness is usually a thirty-minute aerobic workout.

17. Higher Tolerance for Fatigue.

When you're fit, you "hang tougher" under crises.

18. Promotes Clearer and More Rational Thought.

When in shape, you focus on things rationally rather than emotionally. Physical inactivity seems to make the mind go dull. Exercise helps to "clean the static from the attic."

19. Less Clotting of the Blood.

Exercise makes the blood platelets less sticky and less likely to clog.

20. Releases Nature's Tranquilizers (Called Endorphins).

Also called mood elevators, endorphins are responsible for a sense of well-being and the euphoric feeling we experience after a good workout.

The exercise boom is something that would never have happened in a society of farmers and laborers. But with so many bodies expanding due to the mechanization of society and the overwhelming research that excess fat is not healthy, some people realized that exercise had to become part of their daily activity. However, not enough are committed, as almost sixty percent of American adults are sedentary. If it weren't for the fact that the TV and the refrigerator are so far apart, some people wouldn't get any exercise at all. What will hurt future generations the most is that exercise in many schools has neither a presence nor is considered important. Even though the body needs movement, educators place more and more emphasis on the classroom. With fifty percent of America's kids overweight, there is a need to re-assess the decision to eliminate mandatory physical education classes.

Although the aerobic exercise boom was incorrectly and unfortunately classified as a "women's movement" for getting fit, it is, nevertheless, a high-profile activity that is fun and gets a lot more people into working out. Almost every exercise center and cable television station has an aerobics exercise class.

Aerobics is a term attributed to Dr. Kenneth Cooper of Dallas, Texas. In simple terms, it is any exercise which forces the body's larger muscle groups to work repetitively over a period of time. This includes running, walking, swimming, bicycling, rowing, and cross-country skiing. Aerobics is the cornerstone of any fat-burning plan, because fat needs oxygen to burn and provides one with energy. Of all the elements of fitness, the most crucial is cardiovascular fitness.

In exercise, research has shown that moderate intensity is best. High intensity burns sugar, while moderate intensity burns fat. If you start panting, your intensity is too high. Overly intense exercise also tends to suppress your immune system, and there generally are more muscular-skeletal problems associated with very heavy workouts.

As weight and/or fat are lost, the amount of energy expended for the activity decreases. Fewer calories are burned, and subsequent weight/fat loss becomes slower. At that point, you need to increase the intensity of your daily exercises.

The major discrepancy of opinion among aerobics

experts is the time duration for a healthy workout. The time generally ranges from 20–45 minutes. When I went to the YMCA and subsequently lost the two inches, the aerobic portion of the workout was 18–20 minutes. What I have found is that the longer the workout, the tougher it is for busy people to allot the time to faithfully stick with such a program. As well, in exercise there appears to be a point of diminishing return. More is not necessarily better, as too much exercise tends to suppress the immune system. Twenty to thirty minutes seems to be about right. But the key is to do it continuously. Stopping for even one minute allows the heart rate to return to near normal, therefore destroying the aerobic, fat-burning effect. Aerobics require sustained activity.

How often should you exercise? Basically, your current level of fitness is maintained at about three times per week. Therefore, to see improvement you need to work out four to six times per week. Do not feel guilty if you miss the odd day. Aerobic capacity stays for about six weeks before declining.

Aerobic exercise is the best because it is the only activity that gets to the "fat" of the matter. If done correctly, the body will switch from burning carbohydrates as its energy source to burning fat. And remember, as you become more fit, you will need to exercise more vigorously.

Finally, a word here in favor of walking. A brisk walk (about 120 steps per minute) is terrific. It gives you the most health benefits without the risks associated with intense exercise. I recommend you walk your dog every day, even if you don't own a dog.

7.1 Weightlifting and Strength

Strength training is the only way to gain muscle weight. Skip the protein powders and dietary supplements propagating weight gain. They will generally make you gain fat, not muscle, due to high protein and fat content. The optimal fitness program combines aerobic exercises with muscle building. Nobody has died because their muscles weren't big enough, and if you only have time for one activity, then cardiovascular fitness is the more important of the two. However, if time permits, I would highly recommend you include a muscle-building program a few times a week, particularly if you have lost a fair bit of weight and your muscle tone needs improvement. Muscle tone is the tension the muscle holds at rest. Your muscle is metabolically active tissue, and it takes more calories to maintain a muscle and its tone than it does inert fat. Lean muscle provides a furnace for burning fat.

Only exercise builds muscle mass and strength, not food. Carbohydrates give energy, but not bigger or stronger muscles. Generally, women do not have as much muscle mass as men (about two-thirds); however, pound for pound, they are just as strong.

When working the muscles, the weights must be heavy enough to cause complete muscle fatigue after eight or nine repetitions. If you get to fifteen, the weight is too light. The muscle strengthens during the resting state (after lifting weights), not during the exercise itself. Therefore, vary the muscle groups used if you work out on successive days. Generally, strength training two or three times per week will result in the addition of one pound of muscle per month. Anybody who is already physically fit is burning off more calories as they read this book.

Since muscle mass appears to disappear as we get older, it's helpful to do strength training throughout your life, unless you are still working at a job where you are fortunate enough to be exercising your muscles regularly.

7.2   The Athlete

Most of the preceding applies to the athlete, both from a nutritional standpoint and from an exercise standpoint. However, the athlete has a few specific needs and items to be aware of.

First of all, the athlete generally needs extra calories for energy, and this energy should principally come from carbohydrates. Fats are used for long-term endurance. The athlete needs about the same amount of protein as the non-athlete sitting behind the desk. Remember, there is no possibility of increasing muscle mass by eating more protein. Also, a high-fat diet causes blood cells to stick together, thereby decreasing the blood flow. After a high-fat meal, the level of oxygen in your blood drops about twenty percent. This means less oxygen goes to the muscles, which, in turn, limits one's performance. Also, vitamins and minerals are not energy sources, as they act only as catalysts for energy reactions. An athlete's secret to success is not to be found in a pill, bottle, or syringe.

Secondly, selection of the pre-performance meal is critical. It should be a meal that is easy to digest. Otherwise, the energy required to digest the food will detract from the performance. The meal eaten the night before is an important one. Full digestion should be completed prior to competition so that, during competition, the body is using nutrients. Athletes need to drink lots of fluids to replace sweat loss. When I was growing up, we were forbidden to drink water while competing. Because research later proved this only caused dehydration, athletes are now encouraged to take all the water they feel they need.

Oxygen uptake is the ultimate expression of fitness. Oxygen uptake is the amount of oxygen you can take in and use at the cellular level to convert to energy. All athletes should know what their oxygen uptake is.

And finally, training should be strenuous, not abusive.

7.3   Components of Fitness

There are four components of fitness: cardiovascular, muscular endurance, muscular strength, and flexibility.

1. Cardiovascular fitness. Attained through a regular aerobic program, a good cardiovascular system allows you to perform longer, while breathing easily and recovering quickly.

2. Muscular endurance. The ability of muscular groups to respond to prolonged activity, endurance training conditions the body to use more fat as fuel during exercise.

3. Muscular strength. When muscles have to

perform against a load of 75% or more of their potential, more muscle fibers are added. This gives more muscle strength.

4. Flexibility. Stretching enhances flexibility. When you stretch, you free up blood from the stretched muscles. This is equivalent to "letting the offensive units back on the field," thus increasing the efficiency of the immune system.

7.4 Exercise Myths

Myth Number One:

If you have fat on your stomach, sit-ups will take it off. Spot reducing (in other words, exercising the muscle with fat on it) does not work. The fat on your body is deposited in certain areas, but it belongs to the whole body. The only effective way to remove it is by eating a little less fat each day and incorporating an aerobic activity into your life style.

Myth Number Two:

Through exercise, you can convert fat into muscle. It is physiologically impossible for fat tissue to turn into muscle tissue. They are two separate entities.

Myth Number Three:

No pain, no gain. This is an old theory. Pain is not necessary to improve your fitness level. Take the talk test. If you can still carry on a conversation while exercising, you are working at a good pace. Train, but don't strain.

Myth Number Four:

You need more protein for energy when you exercise. Actually, the less protein you eat, the less tired you will be. When you exercise, your body doesn't need more protein; what it does need is more carbohydrates.

Myth Number Five:

Running burns a lot more calories than walking. Actually, both running and walking burn approximately the same amount of calories if you traverse the same distance with equal effort. Walking just takes longer.

Myth Number Six:

Wearing heavy sweat and rubber suits help you lose fat quicker. You do not "sweat off" fat. You metabolize, or "burn," it off. All this extra apparel does is interfere with the body's ability to cool itself.

Myth Number Seven:

When sick, exercise; it will help you get better sooner. When the body is sick, it needs rest. Exercise breaks down the body tissue, so it has to repair and rebuild. When sick, put all your energy into healing. A shorter "sick time" means you will be exercising again sooner.

Myth Number Eight:

It's best to exercise in the morning. Actually, when you exercise is a personal preference. The key is just doing it.

7.5 How to Begin, and Stick with, Your Exercise Program

1. Be PATIENT, but remain consistent and committed. It takes about two to three months to change an old habit (i.e., laziness). Losing fat/weight is not always easy.

2. Write your exercise into your daily planner or on your calendar. You have a personal appointment. DO NOT CANCEL IT. If someone needs you, tell them you are late for an appointment with a pair of running shoes.

3. Begin gradually. The body can handle

a lot of stress, but it should be introduced gradually.

4. Find the right time. Choose a time when you are least likely to have any interruptions.

5. Have some motivating aides. Take a photo (preferably a side shot) of your protruding stomach. For women, take a photo of the back of your thighs. Place these pictures on the re-frigerator, beside the bed, etc. Or carry a picture of your young daughter or son, for whom you want to stick around and watch grow up.

6. Find a partner. It's been proven that if you exercise with a partner versus going it alone, your chances of sticking through it improve from around 10% up to 80%.

7. Vary your routine. Variety helps you psychologically, and it can also prevent overuse injuries which come from pounding away at the same exercise.

8. Keep a chart. We all like to see how we progress. It's our personal score sheet.

9. Do not be obsessed with weight loss alone. In fact, you may lose inches but put on weight, because muscle weighs one and two-tenths more than fat.

10. Even the smallest of movements will help your overall fitness. If you go shopping, park a hundred yards away instead of in the handicapped spot. Or take the stairs instead of the elevator or escalator.

Finding time for exercise starts with your realization of its importance. Commitment is paramount. Lord Derby aptly put it: "If you can't find time for fitness, you'll have to find time for illness."

Fun isn't the point of exercise. It's how good you feel after you've put your body through a good workout. Exercise is truly one of the two pillars of health, nutrition being the other. Its rewards are so great that all physicians should encourage their patients to incorporate regular physical activity into their lives.

Inch, Fat, and Weight Loss

Any successful loss of inches, fat, and weight is ideally accomplished by a change in your food choices, followed by an appropriate exercise program. Because our bodies can store fat in a lot of places we cannot see, we can be getting fat without realizing or feeling it. It isn't until the extra inches appear on our stomachs, hips, or thighs that we become concerned.

Most overweight people choose the wrong foods and combine this with a sedentary lifestyle. From a motivational standpoint, people like to go by weight loss because it usually happens faster than inch loss. The latter occurs so gradually that you don't notice it until one day your clothes feel loose. In this section, I'm going to refer to weight loss, but it will inherently mean fat and inch loss, too.

The physiological goal of weight loss should be to change your body from a "fat storer" to a "fat burner." Muscle burns calories; fat stores them. Any weight loss program must encompass a permanent change in your eating habits. Otherwise, right after you get to your desired weight and pant or dress size, you will start eating the same foods that got you into trouble in the first place. The failure to permanently change your eating habits is the number one reason why 95% of the people gain weight back after they stop the program.

Nutritionally, eliminate most of the protein you eat. Secondly, cut your intake of fats to about ten to fifteen percent of your total calories. Focus on carbohydrates, even though your body will crave fats and refined sugar. Carbohydrates are low in calories and will fill you up sooner, thereby decreasing the desire to eat more.

The second key element in achieving permanent weight loss is boosting your metabolism. This is done through exercise, as it helps to increase muscle mass, which is high-maintenance tissue. The more muscle mass you have, the more calories your body will burn just trying to feed and repair it. There is only one way fat leaves the body: IT MUST BE "BURNED," OR METABOLIZED. And this requires oxygen. This is where an aerobic exercise comes in.

Losing weight quickly is not healthy. Ideally, you should lose one to three pounds per week. Fast weight loss is dangerous, unhealthy, and doesn't last for long unless you have previously altered your eating habits. If you only lost one pound a week for a year, you'd lose fifty-two pounds. To show you how realistic this is, one pound is 3,500 calories. If you just cut out 500 calories a day (7 days times 500 equals 3,500), you would lose one pound a week. By simply eliminating something like your daily milkshake, which is around 500 calories, this can be accomplished. Now, couple this with an exercise program, and you are well on your way. During your weight loss program, there will be periods when you can't seem to break through to the next plateau. Your body is stubbornly hanging on to stay at that weight. It's like the thermostat in your house. At this point, you must not give in to cravings. THIS IS THE CHALLENGE POINT. If you persevere, you will change your body chemistry forever.

Women have an easier time putting on weight externally. They start out with thirteen percent essential fat, whereas men begin with only three percent. You should know your percentage of body fat because it will give you an indication of how over-fat you are. An ideal range would be 10–12% for men and 19–22% for women.

8.1   The Dieting Game

So far, we've talked about how to plan a successful weight loss program, but we should address what most people in the Western world play—the dieting game. It is definitely America's most popular pastime and truly a phenomena of the twentieth century. At any one time in the U.S., approximately forty million people are trying to lose weight. What an anomaly! Rich people are dieting, while poor people are starving.

At the end of a Health and Fitness Seminar in Chicago, a Mr. Harris came up to me with his chart, which showed that he had lost over 300 pounds in the last 10 years—yet now he was fatter and weighed more than he had when he began his first diet program. Each time a new book prophesying the latest scheme to lose weight came out, Mr. Harris would buy it and follow it. None worked. Nor will they ever work—long term. Diets do work, but only in the short term. That is why they are a billion dollar enterprise. Mr. Harris could be on his yo-yo diets forever. When laying out the format for this book, I had originally put dieting under the heading "Diseases of the Affluent," but dieting is not the disease. It's the dependence upon it that is the problem. Dieting is dumb. Here's why.

Shortly after you begin dieting, the body senses an emergency (starvation) and goes into a survival mode. When calories are reduced, the body reacts by slowing down its metabolism so it can hang on to the calories it has. Your metabolic rate can lower as much as twenty pecent in a few weeks. This lowering of metabolism frustrates the dieter, as weight loss will be minimal.

However, if we do lose weight on a diet and do not exercise, we don't just lose fat. If we lose twenty pounds, it would be broken down roughly as follows: ten pounds of fat (good), five pounds of water (okay, if bloated), and five pounds of metabolism-boosting muscle (terrible). Losing five pounds of muscle is what causes dieters to have a "frumpy look," as they lose lean muscle and, ultimately, their body tone. Lean muscle, as we discussed, is the calorie-burning potential of the body. What the body doesn't need is another diet; it needs a faster metabolism.

8.2   Metabolism

Metabolism is the sum of all the chemical processes, or reactions, taking place in your body's organs and cells. It means changing. We all have a base metabolic rate (BMR). This is the amount of energy required to maintain the body's functions when at rest. It is directly proportional to the amount of lean muscle mass in your body. It is higher in males, due to a leaner body mass. It is inherited but can be adjusted by food choices and physical activity. As muscle mass increases, a resting metabolic rate increases.

Muscle tissue is the active tissue of your body. The more muscle you have, the more energy you need and the more calories you burn. It takes about six to eight weeks to increase your metabolic rate. On the other hand, fat cells are less active than other cells. Therefore, the more fat you have in relation to muscle, the lower your metabolic rate. The lower your metabolic rate, the less energy you will burn while resting or exercising.

A study at the Royal Prince Alfred Hospital in Sydney, Australia, pointed out the importance of a high BMR in the burning of calories. It

201

showed the following expenditures: 12% from physical activity, 15% from production of heat, and 73% from BMR. In other words, 73% of our calories are expended by our basic metabolic rate. Therefore, the higher the BMR, the more calories we burn off (without any exercise).

Our BMR is slower at the end of the day and is the slowest during sleep. It is also believed that our metabolic rate slows as we get older, but this may be related to the fact that people are just less active as they age. Another problem is that adults tend to eat the same size portions they consumed as teenagers. Our BMR can also be slowed by our habits. One of the major culprits in slowing BMR is alcohol. When people consume alcohol, their bodies burn fat more slowly than usual. Alcohol suppresses the body's already stingy disposal of fat, and any fat not burned is stored. Swiss researchers found that just six beers lower the body's burning of fat by thirty-three percent (Nutrition and Dietary Consultants, September 1992).

8.3   The Calorie: Friend or Villain?

The calorie can be your friend or a villain. As villain, it is a question of both too little and too much. Without calories (your fuel intake and energy content of food), you would die. With too many calories, you can also die (obesity-related diseases).

Calories equal energy. In simple terms, if you consume more energy (the food you eat) than the energy you expend (movement), your body fat will increase. Today, we have a problem in America because thirty percent of our diet consists of empty calories, calories that make you fat but have no nutritional value. If a product says "high energy" on the label, it usually means high calorie. And remember, all calories are not created equal. It makes a big difference whether the calories are from clean-burning carbohydrates or stick-to-your-waistline fats.

Women generally need fewer calories than men (about twenty-five percent less). Your caloric needs generally decline with age. Therefore, if you eat the same number of calories at age forty as you did at age twenty, you will probably put on weight. Children need more calories than adults (about double the amount) to fuel their growth and high activity level.

One final note: it's not always the food that is the problem. It's what you do with it that piles up the calories. For example, the much-maligned potato is not fattening by itself. A 3.5-ounce potato is about 93 calories. However, when you turn that same potato into french fries, it equals 274 calories. And one step further—turn that potato into potato chips, and you have a whopping 570 calories. The calorie is your friend, but too much of your friend can damage the relationship. We are what we don't get rid of.

In summation, good health must be earned through daily discipline, both in controlling what you eat and in ensuring that you exercise. Proper nutrition, an aerobic exercise, and strength training equals weight and inch loss. You must guard your health as if it were your most precious possession. If you can't take care of yourself, who can you take care of?

Ecological Stewardship

Ecology is the study of how living entities interact with each other and their planetary environment. Stewardship is being in a supervisory capacity.

If one were to grade modern human beings' efforts in taking care of our planet, particularly in the last fifty years, we would definitely receive an "F" for failure. And all are definitely paying the price for altering Mother Nature and pushing her to her limits. The environmental devastations for which we are responsible have global consequences. The world today is in deep peril because the environment has deteriorated as a result of human activity.

Our world has broken apart at an alarming rate for we have failed to appreciate the common bond and link we have to all species. All living entities play an important role and share ecologically—from the smallest bacteria to the earthworm to the human. We should learn how to use the Earth so that her productivity is enhanced rather than diminished. With modern agricultural methods, the latter is what's been happening.

Beginning in the late 1980s, an increased awareness of such crises began among the general population. Schools opened their classrooms to lessons on how to improve and save the environment. But, surprisingly, the most environmentally destructive practice on Earth has been largely overlooked, namely, the killing of animals for food and byproducts.

The meat industry is linked to water, land, and air pollution; deforestation; water shortages; ozone layer depletion; and the global warming trend. As well, soil erosion and consequent desertification turn arable lands into deserts. If you are a meat eater, you are greatly contributing to the destruction of the environment. There isn't a single ecological reality that is not adversely impacted by the meat industry. Our food choices do more to either harm or heal our environment than any other single act.

If there were planetary policemen handing out citations for ecological offenses, meat industries would be paying a lot of fines. Here are the top ten ecological citations:

9.1 Ecological Citations

Citation Number One: An Accomplice in Major Rain Forest Destruction

The rain forests are a 3,000-mile-wide greenbelt that straddles the equator. Rain forests are irreplaceable habitats for approximately half of the world's plants and animals. They are our richest and most diverse biological treasure. They recycle and purify our water and play an essential role in the generation of weather around the planet. In the 1970s and 1980s, rain forests were being destroyed for the grazing of cattle at the rate of a football field every five seconds, or an area the size of Denmark every six months. Forests are leveled to make way for pastures by the 100,000 cattle ranchers in Amazonia alone. Large food corporations bought hundreds of miles of rain forests in Amazonia; those lands are being destroyed for only a privileged few.

The roots of the trees in a rain forest are very superficial, and the soil is nutrient-poor for growing food for human consumption. Therefore, after the cattle have finished grazing, the land is stripped and is no longer suitable for agriculture or rain forest regrowth. So, the ranchers move on, burning and slashing more and more of this treasured land.

Rain forests continue to be decimated so that more hamburgers can be produced. Christopher Uhl, Assistant Professor of Biology at Penn State, guesstimates that one hamburger costs fifty-five square feet of rain forest (the USDA says seventy-eight square feet)—a debt never to be repaid. The large amounts of most beef produced in Central and South America are not consumed there, but are shipped to the U.S. and Europe for consumption. Imported South American "rain forest beef" is but a small amount of America's total beef consumption. But exports to the U.S., Europe, and other industrialized countries are a very large percentage of the South American beef trade.

This trading of forests for hamburgers

displaces both animal and human life. The indigenous tribes, whose ecological wisdom greatly surpasses ours, are forced to move into towns and cities. Their knowledge is invaluable and can save our lives, as the rain forests also contain our future medicines. Modern societies see them as primitive people. Ecologically and environmentally sensitive people see them as great sages.

And what about flooding? Whenever trees are destroyed, the damage to the natural environment is almost irreversible. We end up with a landscape that cannot hold water. Consequent flooding destroys homes and displaces families.

The hamburger rose to prominence at the expense of the native people of other countries, especially those in Central and South America. Costa Rica was almost completely cloaked in tropical rain forests, yet it's been sacrificed for meat production. Local people don't consume the food, as almost all of the meat is exported. The cattle ranchers are more interested in short-term profit than long-term conservation. South American beef may be cheap to some wealthy countries, but it's extremely expensive in terms of ecological consequences and the economic well-being of common people. Prosperous nations have no right expanding their so-called luxury at the expense of poorer nations.

I know it's hard to worry about something that is so far away and is in someone else's backyard, but your help is needed. Rain forests are essential to all human activity, and the survival of the remaining rain forests will greatly impact our personal lives in the future. Our eating habits threaten all rain forests, and you can help right now by making wise food choices.

The 1990s may be the last chance we have to preserve the valuable rain forest. The ecological literacy of media reporters worldwide needs to be enhanced so they can, in turn, educate the general population about the environmental effects of cattle consumption.

Citation Number Two: Aiding in the Rapid Extinction of Species

In researching this section, I found an extreme set of numbers representing the species currently becoming extinct each year as we continue to rape precious land. The smallest number per year was 1,000 and the largest was 150,000. Even if we were to take the lowest number, it is too many and far, far above the rate of extinction that would occur naturally without the intervention of destructive human beings. The slash-and-burn forest clearing of cattle ranchers has condemned countless species to extinction. Species that lose their homes are often incapable of adjusting to a new habitat.

What causes the increase in the number of

species becoming extinct? It is due to the fact that there is full interdependence of species in the kingdom of the rain forest. What is waste to one creature is essential to another for survival. Environmentally sensitive individuals do a lot of composting, returning materials to the land. This is nature's way of regeneration. When we kill one species, we upset the delicate balance of the ecosystem.

For example, frogs' legs became very popular to export a few decades ago in countries such as India, Bangladesh, and China, which were feverishly trading in frogs for consumption around the world. They were forced to scale back dramatically when the mosquito population got out of control, for frogs eat and control mosquitoes. With more mosquitoes, malaria started killing millions of people again.

So, the next time you wonder what the purpose and value of a particular species are, remember that no species exists without both supporting and being supported by another species of life.

Citation Number Three: Failing to Replace Topsoil

Topsoil is the most basic foundation of our existence on Earth. It is the dark, nutrient-rich soil that holds moisture and feeds us by feeding the plants. It is our ultimate lifeline. Every great nation has risen or fallen according to the quality of its topsoil. Topsoil depletion has caused the demise of many great civilizations. The Sahara Desert, once a fertile range land and rich land mass, continues to move south at a rate of thirty miles per year.

Billions of tons of topsoil in America are eroded yearly due to animal agriculture. John Robbins, in his book *Diet for a New America*, says that "Eighty-eight percent of our topsoil erosion is due to livestock production." In the last 200 years, we've lost 75% of our topsoil, and it takes 100–500 years to regain just one inch of topsoil.

The disappearance of our topsoil is caused in two principal ways. The first is when land is cleared for grazing. The removal of trees triggers erosion due to the loss of soil stability. Secondly, the hooves of heavy cattle compact the land, squeezing out air. This means that the land is less able to absorb water and keep it moist for future growth. The once valuable, now hardened land dries out and blows away. These dust bowls become an accomplice in flooding. You don't have to be a farmer to recognize the urgency to curb depletion of our topsoil.

Citation Number Four: Polluting and Mismanaging the Land

An enormous amount of land would be freed if we stopped using it for animal agriculture. The

USDA says that fifty percent of available land is used to raise livestock, while only four percent is used for growing fruits and vegetables. How did things get so out of balance? Eighty to ninety percent of our grain is fed to livestock that is later killed for meat. What a waste of land that could have been used to grow food for direct human consumption!

How much more fruit and vegetable produce could have been grown on land that is currently used for livestock! The USDA says that an acre of land, which can yield approximately 20,000 pounds of potatoes, yields only about 165 pounds of beef. And all of this continues to go on, while over one billion people globally are categorized as "starving." We need to free our land so that it may grow food for human consumption instead of feed for livestock.

The meat industry is the number one polluter. John Robbins calculates that 50,000 pounds of animal excrement per second go into our land and waterways. Most of the vast cattle feed lots do not have sewage disposal systems.

Modern agriculture is big business. It is profit-based and has destroyed the majority of small farms in America. Many farms are now single-crop entities. This is bad for the land, which works best if crops are rotated.

With this big business, we have become the first civilization to grow food with poisons (i.e., pesticides). "Pesticide" is an umbrella term for herbicides, insecticides, and fungicides. If you eat food produced in the U.S., you probably eat pesticides. Chemical presence in our foods today is so pervasive that trying to avoid them is almost physically impossible. We are taking goodness from the Earth and replacing it with poison. Millions and millions of species at the bottom of the food chain are being poisoned to death.

Fortunately, with fruits, grains, and vegetables, we can clean much of the pesticide spray off the surface; however, we cannot remove the pesticides deposited in animal fat. All animal food is high on the food chain, and animals are subjected to the highest levels of environmental contaminates. And when humans eat it, they are the recipients of this pesticide residue. This is why organically grown fruits, vegetables, and grains are increasingly more popular.

According to the Environmental Protection Agency (EPA), 70,000 chemicals are being used today, and the pesticides used in farming do not necessarily kill the intended victims. They just end up polluting our land and water. Resistance to any foreign substance is natural to evolution. Bugs, insects, and parasites develop a resistance to chemicals when they are exposed to a concentrated amount that doesn't kill them. And what does modern agriculture do? Tries another chemical. And the cycle continues.

Today, insects kill as many crops as they did before the mass introduction of chemicals. Chemicals never solved the problem—they just poisoned our food.

Citation Number Five: Water Depletion and Pollution

Our waterways have become nothing more than mixtures of highly toxic substances. Many former pristinely pure rivers and lakes have either died or are now on the verge of biological death. The sewage from factory farms is the biggest water polluter associated with animal agriculture. Feed lots and slaughterhouses are not only the major polluters of our water (with sewage and pesticides), but they also use up a majority of our fresh drinking water. An article in *Newsweek* pointed out that the water needed to produce a 1,000-pound steer could float a destroyer. Jeremy Rifkin, in his book *Beyond*

Beef, estimates that seventy percent of all water consumed goes to animal feed and food.

I remember being at a restaurant in Monterey, California, in 1990, and noticing that water was not placed on our table shortly after we were seated. I found out that it was against the law. The only way you could get a glass of water was to request it. The guy at the next table was able to eat his steak, yet nobody thought or calculated how much water it had taken to get it to his table. (Note: It takes approximately 3,500 gallons of water to produce one pound of meat, whereas 60 gallons of water can produce a pound of wheat.)

And what about the enormous amounts of water needed to irrigate the land to grow food for the animals right up until the final act, when water is needed to dispose of the animal's excrement following the slaughter? What's worse is that the government subsidizes this water use—all for food that ultimately becomes our number one killer. In addition, pesticide runoff is a major polluter of our water; once these toxins enter our waterways, they are very difficult to get out.

Without water, we are history in seven to ten days. Even one day without water is unhealthy. It's so important to our future that we can no longer sit back and allow our waterways to be an indiscriminate dumping ground. Becoming a vegetarian contributes more toward cleaning and preserving our water than any other single act.

Citation Number Six: Air Pollution

The meat industry receives a citation for air pollution because of its failure to replace the trees on the land it has used. There is no question they could be cited for the irreversible use (and waste) of energy involved in the transport of animals to slaughterhouses thousands of miles every day (sixteen million miles per day in the U.S. alone). It takes an estimated ten times the amount of energy to transport animals as it does vegetables. And what about the dependence on tractors, which guzzle fossil fuels?

It is also worth pointing out that the largest source of particulate air pollution by far is the hundreds of millions of tons of topsoil that blow off American farmlands every year. Of all industries, the meat industry, by allowing its cattle to graze and then move on, is by far the most insensitive to our ecosystem and land.

Trees are one of the principal "pollution control units" of this planet. We live in harmony with trees. We inhale oxygen and exhale carbon dioxide (CO_2). Trees absorb CO_2 and release oxygen. The cycle is complete. The more plant life we have, the more carbon dioxide is taken from the air and replaced with oxygen.

Today, however, we are increasing the

amount of CO_2 released into the air (from car exhaust and dead, burning, and rotting trees), while decreasing our forest population of plants. Anyone who has been to Singapore recently has probably noticed the improvement in their air quality, which can be directly attributed to the energetic planting of millions of trees in the city. In addition, trees can process forty gallons of moisture and release it into the air—the resulting rain cleans the air.

One of the best contributions one can make to offset this dramatic loss of part of our ecosystem is to plant trees or other plants. In addition, trees create new soil, supply nutrients to the land, keep the soil moisturized by drying up ground water, and bind the soil to protect it from wind and soil erosion. They are our best partners in helping to heal our planet.

If we don't begin cleaning up our air, we'll have to put oxygen on our shopping list. Sound far-fetched? Bottled water in stores would have sounded strange to people in 1900 as well.

Citation Number Seven: Contributing to Global Warming

In addition to polluting the air, the meat industry is a big contributor to global warming, which is attributed to the greenhouse effect. Global warming occurs when certain chemicals trap heat from the Earth's surface, preventing it from escaping into space. *Time* magazine, in its January 2, 1989 issue, explained this as follows: "Like panes of glass of a greenhouse, the CO_2 molecules are transparent to visible light, allowing the sun's rays to warm the Earth's surface. But when the Earth's surface gives off extra heat, it does so with infrared radiation. Since CO_2 absorbs infrared rays, some of the excess heat stays in the atmosphere."

Almost fifty percent of global warming is

caused by CO_2. CO_2 is important, as we need to trap some warmth. Otherwise, the sun would merely reflect off the Earth. It is the unprecedented amounts being released (about a thirty percent increase since 1900) that are dangerous. When cattle ranchers burn the rain forest, millions of tons of carbon dioxide are spewed into the atmosphere, magnifying the greenhouse effect.

Excess methane can be more dangerous, as it traps 20–25 times the amount of CO_2 (molecule for molecule). It is released whenever organic matter breaks down. Both termites and cattle have, in their guts, microorganisms that digest cellulose and produce methane. We have too many artificially produced cattle on the planet (approximately 1.4 billion in 1992) that are belching and flatulating, thus releasing methane (about 12–20% of the total methane). Termites that cut down forests are thriving, as their populations increase in dead forests (they can lay up to 10,000 eggs a day).

Flooded rice paddies are among the sources of methane as well. As ocean temperatures rise due to global warming, there will be more flooding of low-lying lands. Also predicted are more violent hurricanes and significantly altered weather patterns. And, most importantly, higher temperatures cause droughts—a potential disaster for our food supply.

Citation Number Eight: Contributing to the Depletion of the Ozone Layer

The ozone layer is located 12–20 miles from Earth's surface. It is Earth's protective shield— a thin, natural filter of the sun's harmful rays. A hole in the shield was discovered by British scientists in Antarctica in the mid-1980s. Ozone depletion is linked to a rapid rise in skin cancer (especially in Australia, so near Antarctica and with a predominantly white population). The principal contributors to opening holes in the ozone layer are CO_2 and methane. Others are:

1. CFC's (chloro-fluorcarbons). These are the most dangerous because they are so durable and are about 20,000 times as efficient at trapping as one molecule of CO_2. They are found in freezers, air conditioners, and Styrofoam containers. Our dependence on the freezer is the result of our dependence on meat, chicken, and fish, which have to be kept cool to prevent rapid decay. And even though they are being phased out, far too many hamburgers were served in throw-away, Styrofoam containers.

2. Oxides of nitrogen. These principally come from auto exhaust. Can we repair the holes? Yes. Every lightning bolt makes ozone, and ozone makes ozone. But before we put the onus on nature to once again repair, we must take responsibility ourselves

by stopping our contribution to making the holes bigger.

The sunshine, filtered through the ozone layer, is our friend. The sun is a great detoxifier. It opens up our pours and releases toxins through our skin, and it has an enormous effect on our moods. Research has shown that patients on the sunny side of a hospital make quicker recoveries. And anyone who has stepped outside on a bright, sunny day has experienced a wonderful sense of well-being. We must close the hole, and you now know how you can contribute.

Citation Number Nine: Destroying and Endangering Future Medicines

When cattle ranchers began their massive destruction of rain forests, probably none of them gave a single thought to the fact that they were destroying plants that do and will supply us with valuable medicines. The rain forests are a rich pool of plant life with medicinal benefits. Yet these plants are threatened with extinction at the hands of multinational corporations and wealthy cattle ranchers. We need to respect these ancient, irreplaceable nurseries of life. The Amazon is truly the greatest "pharmaceutical lab." Cancer is rampant, and the National Cancer Institute points out that seventy percent of the plants that have anti-cancer properties come from the tropical rain forest.

Citation Number Ten: Insensitivity to Life—Human, Animal, and Plant

Hunger follows cattle ranchers. And the ranchers continue to meet our demands for the flesh that humans eat in such large quantities. The world's poor end up with devastated homelands that cannot be farmed. A small elite in third world countries have sold their ecological souls.

Almost every pound of animal flesh is produced at the expense of a burning rain forest or an eroded range land. Wildlife habitat is destroyed to create cattle pastures, and this reverberates around the world. When birds lose their homes, they often die. Fewer birds mean more insects. More insects means more pesticide use, which means even fewer birds, as many die from these poisons.

And what about the ultraviolet rays killing ocean phytoplankton because of the ozone hole? Phytoplankton form the base of the oceanic food chain, as well as provide a significant amount of the world's oxygen. Without phytoplankton, most life forms would suffocate. We kill this, and we kill our oceans.

Rain forest populations do not adapt well to human invasion. There is enough information at hand now for us to stop. Any further use of land for cattle ranching is a conscious decision, based on short-term profit instead of a long-term concern—not only for our well-being but also the well-being of our children and their children. This insensitivity is augmented by ranchers and their customers treating animals as commodities instead of sentient beings with faces, families, and feelings.

Jeremy Rifkin writes in *Beyond Beef*, "There is a curious silence surrounding the issue of cattle being one of the most destructive environmental threats." We need to break the silence, as we may be the last generation with the chance to save our environment.

In summation, we have created an environmental and ethical disaster. The rapid destruction and extinction of our valuable natural resources, which will be needed for future generations, is an unparalleled crime. Our dependence on meat, chicken, and fish has resulted in a huge environmental toll—from the rain forest to factory farms to the drift nets. This destruction process has been wholly engineered by the human population, and it's up to us to deal with the consequent environmental urgency for repair.

The world's environmental problems will not be solved until we cut back on our overwhelming desire for material consumption. There was a time when our air was clean, our rivers ran pure, and the multitude of birds made the world a lot more musical.

The Moral Perspective

This chapter was the most difficult for me to write. First of all, I feel it is the most important, and secondly, it was difficult to not let my emotions overpower the content of this chapter. And when we discuss moral perspectives, there are always the issues of culture and interpretation.

Since external culture can be just another reason to hang on to an old habit, we need to focus on our inner compass. In other words, what our heart tells us.

Compassion is an admirable quality we should all strive to incorporate into our character. Unfortunately, eating meat extinguishes the spark of compassion. Buddha taught that "Unless it eventuates in compassion, knowledge is worthless."

One of the most vital components of compassion is a reverence for life. We must realize that animals have an inherent right to exist, just as we do. Unfortunately, in our modern society we view other creatures as a means to our fulfillment. We snuff out their lives whenever it suits our purpose. Leonardo DaVinci put this in perspective: "He who does not value life does not deserve it." And Albert Schweitzer said, "From the time they start school, young people must be imbued with the idea of reverence for all living things. Then we will be able to develop a spirit based on ethical responsibility and one that will stir many. Then we will be entitled to call ourselves a humanity of culture."

How did we come to accept the high level of cruelty toward animals that is so prevalent today?

Basically, it stems from culture, deception, and selfishness. We often hear: "But people always ate meat." To which you can reply: "But people have always murdered." One doesn't make the other acceptable.

The part of culture that people cling most to are religious scriptures and doctrines. This is such a complex issue—and a book in itself. I refer you to Steven Rosen's *Diet for Transcendence* to evaluate how religious scriptures have been misinterpreted to suit our food choices. Although ancient religions teach a reverence for life and that animals have souls, some of the more modernized religions in the last few thousand years have separated man and animal. The eating of animals has become so commonplace in many countries that it is considered civilized human behavior.

The theory that animals have no souls is simply the theological justification of those who are not interested in animals. People engage in word jugglery in order to rationalize a habit or desire. There is no scriptural basis for this, just as there was no scriptural basis for what was once a popular notion that women didn't have souls. Actually, it's quite the contrary. In all bona fide religions, the animal has a soul. Some of the more modern versions, which do not acknowledge this, are simply tampered translations. All I can say is: How did we drift so far as to think that heaven might be "heaven" at all without animal companionship?

Deception has played a major role in allowing us to develop the flesh habit. We are able to swallow it because we put the cruelty of it out of our minds. How often does one hear, "Don't tell me about the horrific conditions in a slaughterhouse or about what is in my meat, as you will ruin my dinner."

In addition to deceiving ourselves, we are also

greatly deceived by the marketing and public relations machines of the food giants. They use words like "processed" instead of "killed" or "gutted"; "aged" instead of "decomposed or "rotted"; "hamburger" instead of "ground up parts of cow"; and "veal" instead of "tortured baby animal." Ham, bacon, meat, and hot dogs are all deceptive words to cover up reality. And government doesn't help by excluding animals for human consumption in the Animal Welfare Act, which governs the humane treatment of animals.

Finally, we are just plain selfish (and stubborn). We keep a tenacious grip on what we like to eat. Even our intelligence is not a strong enough force at times. Look at how many people know the ill effects of smoking cigarettes and eating meat. They have all the reasons to quit, but they either can't or won't. This is why I feel that unless we add a moral perspective to our food choices, we shall almost always slide backward on our commitment to eating well.

In the big picture, eating well for ourselves is still a selfish motive. We need to broaden our sphere of concern and contribution. Nowhere is there a better focus to understand the increasingly violent nature of people today. How long is it going to take before we make the connection? People who respect animal life have little or no inclination for violent acts against humans. Perhaps one of the greatest ironies occurred at George Bush's Presidential Inauguration. He genuinely talked about a gentler, kinder world. Yet that evening, veal—the product of a very violent industry—was the entríe at dinner.

A powerful approach to opening our hearts is to change places with the creatures whom we abuse and ultimately kill. Experience the pain of a lobster burning to death in boiling water. Or a whale with a harpoon exploding

239

in its side. Or the live puppies in Taiwanese restaurants, soon to end up on a plate. Or the cow in a slaughterhouse, whose throat will be slit while fully conscious because it has to be kosher. Or the mother elephant in Africa, killed so her tusks can be used in billiard balls. Or the trapped animal, about to finally die, so its fur can ultimately ornament somebody.

While in China in the late 1980s, I saw the most insensitive, shocking site when it comes to food choices. Certain tables in the restaurant had holes about three to four inches in diameter in the centers of them. The tables open and close around this hole. A live monkey is brought to the table, which closes around its neck so that only the head is visible. The diners crack open the monkey's skull, pour boiling hot water over it, and consume the brain matter with chopsticks. Horrific scenes with comparable cruelty like this go on every day in America—only they're done behind closed doors.

The award for insensitivity to the animal world would definitely go to tuna fishermen. Since dolphins and tuna tend to swim together, whenever dolphins are sighted, the tuna nets are lowered in the area. Since this method began, a guesstimate is that five million dolphins have been killed. When one dolphin is trapped, the others will stay to give comfort, often singing to him or her. They stay, even if it means also dying. We humans could learn a lot about loyalty from our dolphin friends.

These intelligent, compassionate, sensitive creatures are often referred to as the "people of the sea." So many individuals literally owe their lives to the dolphin for having saved them—and we repay the dolphin by drowning them. They have no record of ever having harmed humans. In fact, experiments have

241

been done in which dolphins were provoked into attacking a human, and they wouldn't do it.

Fortunately, a gentleman by the name of Sam LaBudde went out on a fishing vessel, the *Maria Luisa,* and with a hidden video camera taped the slaughter. Sam was stunned by what he saw and said afterward, "I was spiritually crippled because I was having a difficult time believing and accepting that human beings could be so indifferent to the fate of a species—especially dolphins." We owe these magnificent fellow travelers the right-of-way in their own domain. Leonardo DaVinci wrote, "Truly man is king of the beasts, for our cruelty exceeds theirs."

And our cruelty doesn't end with our food choices. We put a legal stamp on it and call it a sport. George Bernard Shaw put these sports in perspective with the following: "When a man wants to kill an animal, he calls it 'sport.'

When a criminal wants to kill a human, it's called 'ferocity.' If hunting is a sport, ask the deer." It's an anomaly in our society that you can legally shoot and kill a deer who is doing absolutely nothing to harm you, yet it's illegal in thirty states to yell and scare the deer away so it might live.

When I played a tennis tour in Spain, the players were invited to a bullfight. This was before I had become a vegetarian, and at the time I certainly wasn't too sensitive to what happened to animals. But I was shocked at what went on in the ring. I found myself cheering for the bulls the entire time. And they call this a sport, where 30,000 bulls a year are put through a torturous last hour of their lives in front of a stadium of people who find it all very entertaining.

Over the years, we all hear stories or experience acts of kindness or a lack thereof, or maybe we hear a motivational phrase. Whatever the case, these have an impact. I would like to share a few of those with you now.

Story A: In the movie *Dances with Wolves*, they use the Lakota language. In this language, there isn't a word for "animal" because the animals are regarded as brothers or sisters.

Story B: In 1856 Japan, U.S. Ambassador Townsend Harris landed in Tokyo for a press conference. He was accustomed to eating steaks, and he ordered one for dinner. In those days, the Japanese hardly ate meat. However, the host reluctantly complied to having a cow slaughtered to appease the hungry ambassador. To this day, there stands a memorial to that cow.

Story C: In 1987, in Buffalo, New York, a Mr. Michael Halsey was jailed for thirty days for killing a ten-week-old puppy. He was the first person to ever receive such a sentence for the death of a domesticated animal. Judge Michael

Broderick sentenced him for "the killing of a living creature."

Story D: In 1988, I watched a documentary on TV in New Zealand. It was about the lamb industry. There was a gentleman being interviewed who boasted that his plant had killed twenty million lambs. He concluded his comments with, "That's something to be damned proud of."

Story E: A business associate of mine (and former hunter) related one day why he had given up hunting. He had taken his seven-year-old daughter with him. After collecting the bird he had blasted out of the sky, his daughter noticed that the bird still had food in its mouth. When the daughter asked why, he replied, "It was probably carrying the food home to its kids." Whereupon his daughter responded in shock, "Dad, did you shoot someone's parent?"

Story F: My favorite. Ingrid Newkirk, who now heads up People for the Ethical Treatment of

Animals, used to work at an animal shelter. The night before the animals were to be destroyed, she took the scruffiest, ugliest and most decrepit ones for a special meal and a long walk, and basically made a big fuss over them. For most of them, this was the best night of their lives.

When the moral issue of killing animals for food is discussed, there are two common questions I receive. The first is: Aren't plants living entities also? (Many people believe they have souls, so why kill them?) This is a thoughtful question that is best answered in an ancient text, the *Bhagavad-gita,* which states that there is karma (reaction) for all killing. Therefore, you must first offer your food to God to avoid getting a reaction. And God only receives fruits, grains, vegetables, and dairy products. If you are not comfortable with this, remember that most of the food obtained from fruits, grains, vegetables, and dairy products can be obtained without killing the plant or animal. The second question relates to the statement that we have "dominion" over animals. Dominion is the right to rule with sovereign power, not the right to kill. Dominion comes from the same root as domestic, meaning "in your house." Animals are really guests in our home.

Children begin life respecting animals. Just look at a child's crib—it's full of toy animals. A child actually feels much closer to the animal world than to the mysterious adult world. Animals are very much a part of the mental landscape for children. They are attracted to animals like magnets. Children are appalled when they find out we are eating a cuddly lamb or Elsie the cow. But parents do their best to tell them it's okay. Besides, they need their protein.

We all love animals. In fact, more people in America visit zoos than all other sporting events combined. We love to read about animals. *Black Beauty*, written by Anna Sewel in 1877, has sold over thirty million copies. We bring animals into our homes and let them sleep on our beds. We live a dichotomous life, as we pet our dog with one hand and shovel a piece of cow into our mouths with the other.

Dr. Albert Schweitzer put the moral issue into perspective when he said, "To the man who is truly ethical, all of life is sacred. Until man extends his circle of compassion to all living things, he will never find himself in peace." And if the animals could speak, they would say, "Thanks for caring."

And, finally, George Bernard Shaw said, "My will contains directions for my funeral, which will be followed not by mourning coaches, but by herds of oxen, sheep, swine, flocks of poultry, and a small traveling aquarium of live fish, all wearing white scarves in honor of the man who

Quick Tips / Quick Read

Over years of study and personal experience in 134 countries, I have learned a number of tips that have been helpful. They are a potpourri of ideas, thoughts, and suggestions and have no particular order of importance. Some have been briefly discussed in the book so far.

1. Avoid Drinking Fluids with Meals.
Why? It dilutes the digestive juices.

2. Incorporate a Daily Nap into Your Lifestyle.
All societies, up and until the Industrial

Revolution, took an afternoon nap or siesta. Your body craves rest about eight hours after waking up in the morning. A fifteen to twenty-minute nap has been proven to increase alertness and performance. Anything longer makes one wake up dull and groggy. Experts say a short nap in the afternoon actually leaves you more rested than the same amount of time tacked onto the morning sleep. Lying down and resting can be just as restorative.

3. Know Your Prime Time Alertness.

Each of us has a particular time of day when we are at our most productive. Know it so you can do your toughest, most creative tasks during that period.

4. Do Not Eat When Sick.

When sick, we usually lose our appetite. Save your energy for healing and recuperation.

5. Avoid Eating After 6:00 pm As Much As Possible.

In the U.S., we consume about sixty percent of our calories after 6:00 pm, and we don't have much time to burn them off. Eating late at night makes you fat, as your metabolic rate is slower. Eat lighter dinners, and you will notice a difference in your weight and the quality of your sleep. Let your body focus on nerve regeneration rather than digestion, both of which are diminished in the evening.

6. Don't Eat Quickly.

Allow twenty minutes to finish each meal. It takes twenty minutes to feel full. To slow down, try to never have a utensil in your hand while food is in your mouth.

7. Laugh.

The average child laughs or smiles four hundred times a day, the average adult only fifteen times a day. People who do not laugh contract more sickness.

8. Make Lunch Your Biggest Meal.

Lunch was originally called "dinner." Ayurvedic medicine (the original medicine of the world) says the optimal time for best digestion is from 10:00 am–2:00 pm.

9. Always Walk After a Meal.

This greatly increases abdominal blood flow.

10. Don't Sit For Long Periods.

Sitting puts 1 1/2 times the amount of stress on the back as standing, and the blood flow decreases to the unused muscles. Walk a lot on airplane flights. Avoid chairs wherever possible. There are virtually no back problems in India, as they squat or sit cross-legged most of the time.

11. Buy Comfortable Shoes.

During the average lifetime, a pair of feet will walk around the world three times.

12. At the First Sign of Infection, Increase Fluids Tremendously.

This helps your body flush out the bacteria.

13. A Fever Is Your Friend.

When you're sick, fever has a purpose. It makes it tough for germs to reproduce. Unless it's above 103 degrees or if you are terribly uncomfortable, let the fever run its course.

14. Avoid All Focused Work 30–60 Minutes Before Bedtime.

When you lie down in bed, your mind has also begun to wind down, making it easier to fall asleep sooner.

15. Experiment With Two Meals a Day.

You will probably find yourself with a lot more energy.

16. Whenever Your Eyes Begin to Tire or Burn, Stop and Focus on Something in the Distance.

When you look at the horizon, your eye muscles relax.

17. Treat Yourself to Massages.

Ideally, once a day, particularly hands and feet. As well, neck and shoulders—remember, your head weighs around twenty pounds. Massage also helps move the blood and toxins that may have pooled in your body.

18. Avoid Eating If Upset.

For maximum digestion, mealtime should be calm.

19. Take Hot Baths.

Hot baths are good because you submerge yourself in water which is hotter than your body temperature (98.6 degrees). If you start an artificial fever by taking a hot bath, many toxins can be eliminated through the 96 million pours in the skin.

20. Chew, Chew, Chew Your Food.

Slow down. Chew 30–40 times. Chewing also helps eliminate intestinal gas. Fast eaters usually have gas because they take in a lot of air. Chewing forces the air out of food. Chew it long enough to savor and liquefy it.

21. Try Eating Only Fruits for Breakfast.

Since digestion takes more energy than any other function, eat fruits in the morning. Fruits require very little digestive energy.

22. Drink Lots of Water (About 8–10 Glasses a Day).

Give yourself a regular "internal bath."

23. Brush Your Skin with a Loofa Brush.

Skin is often referred to as the "third kidney." It helps clean out the 7–8 million sweat and oil-secreting glands found in the skin.

24. Build Yourself a Garden, Even a Small One.

Gardening is very therapeutic. It puts you in touch with nature. A recent Harris poll found that Americans reported gardening as their favorite form of recreation.

25. Sow an Act of Kindness.

Do something nice for someone, particularly an older person. Their appreciation will make you feel good as well.

26. When Flying, Drink Extra Amounts of Water or Juice.

The air in the cabin of an aircraft is very dry, sometimes drier than a desert. You lose a lot of fluid through dehydration. Therefore, drink lots of water or juice before, during, and after the flight. Avoid caffeine and alcohol, which increase fluid loss.

27. Do Not Overeat in Foreign Countries.

If you eat small amounts, your body's defenses can usually handle the foreign bacteria. Most of the people who get sick in foreign countries do so after eating a big meal.

28. Do Not Soak Your Vegetables in Water After You Cut Them.

You'll lose the water-soluble vitamins.

29. Exercise and Enrich Your Brain, No Matter What Your Age.

The National Institute on Aging pointed out that there is no difference in the brain activity of a healthy man between the ages of 21 and 83. The development of brain cells continues into old age. Regardless of age, nerve cells grow in response to intellectual enrichment. Senility is not a companion of old age if you take care of your health.

30. Watch a Sunset by Water's Edge Alone.

Take some quiet time for yourself. Meditation time is one of the most potent medicines we have.

The Transition

Whenever a life style is altered, there are some hurdles. If you are pretty much convinced that you would like to switch to a vegetarian diet, I would like to share with you some ideas and thoughts that will help ease the transition for you. How dramatic that transition is depends on how you would like to change. Some people are so well disciplined that they can change overnight. You have seen smokers who one day decided to quit, and that was it. They never returned. And then there are others who have to quit ten times before they finally quit for good.

If you stop eating meat, fish, poultry, and

eggs all at one time, there will probably be a few tough days as your body adjusts. You may experience periods of tiredness, headaches, and/or weakness. This is normal, as your body is detoxifying. It finally has a chance to clean out all the garbage you've shoveled into it for years. Remember that animal flesh contains a lot of irritants and stimulants. If these periods come, just slow down a bit and rest. Drink lots of water and juices and eat some fruit. For almost everybody who has done a full transition these periods are brief, lasting only a few days. Then the turnaround begins and you are amazed by how good you feel.

If you are the type of person who likes to transition gradually, the order of food elimination that most people follow is red meat, white meat, fish, and eggs (then dairy products if they switch to a vegan diet). The transitions should be made at a pace that is appropriate for you.

Whatever approach you take, the best advice I could give you is to read up on the subject. You're going to get a lot of questions, challenges, and advice. When I switched in 1970, almost everybody assured me that disease and death would be following soon. Looking back, I am amazed at the advice I received. Not only was it highly inaccurate, but it was the passion with which people gave it. I now understand that it was a combination of fear of the unknown and a justification for them to cling to their old eating habits. The only argument for eating meat, fish, poultry, and eggs is that they taste good. If you can control the three inches of your tongue (where your taste buds are located), you'll do fine. If you have an intellectual and moral understanding of your decision, keeping your commitment will be much easier.

It helps to understand also that a vegetarian diet is completely natural. It is not a diet of deprivation; it is not a sacrifice—but, rather, the acquisition of a new consciousness. It is not a dangerous food choice, as it can provide all nutrients necessary for good health. The word itself comes from the Latin word *vigitore,* which means "giving strength and health." If you ask a vegetarian why they have chosen that lifestyle, you will almost always get a thoughtful, sensible, sensitive answer. On the other hand, if you ask a meat eater why they eat meat, the answers are very shallow: "I like it," "Protein," "It makes me strong."

Fortunately, attitudes toward vegetarianism have changed dramatically. In the early 70s, I was constantly challenged about my new food choices. By the mid-80s, almost every question was one of genuine interest. Almost everybody would say, "I'm gradually changing, too," or "I've changed." (One is no longer considered a "hippie" or a "weirdo" if they are a vegetarian.)

One area of support I feel will be essential in the future is that of the medical profession. Although preventive medicine does not generate nearly as much income as curing, doctors have an obligation. Vegetarianism is definitely the most effective diet in preventing heart diseases, and many are still not saying this.

Support also from your family and friends can be very helpful. Ideally, if all people living under the same roof transition together, it will facilitate the meal preparation. However, if one member refuses to go along, make sure they know how to cook. Seriously, though, this can be a problem. The two solutions that seem to work best are to prepare meals that are both tasty and meatless or have the person eat their "meat meals" at work.

For many people, preparing tasty, meatless meals may sound difficult, but the key is to think ETHNIC. All ethnic foods (Indian, Mexican,

Thai, Italian, Chinese, etc.) were vegetarian in the beginning. Only as their societies became more affluent or Westernized did meat make its way into the menu. In addition, there are many health food stores that sell "fake meat." This is textured vegetable protein that is made to taste like the real thing. For example, you could have spaghetti and meatballs, whereby the "meat eater" in your family would never know the difference. This satisfies their taste buds, and both of you will improve your health. For those of you who like to cook, at the back of the book I have included some of the more popular vegetarian cookbooks.

Traveling and maintaining healthy food choices poses a problem for some people. All that is required is to be a little better organized. For example, when booking your airline flight, you can request a vegetarian meal (a minimum 24-hour advance notice is generally needed).

Granted, some airlines haven't progressed beyond a salad and a plate of vegetables, but some are getting better. Their popularity has increased, as most of the major airlines served over four million vegetarian meals in 1995. Hotel menus are still the worst for vegetarians. I've stayed in hotels for 250–300 days a year for almost thirty years, and I haven't found more than ten hotels that have a decent selection and quality of vegetarian food. But that will change. In the meantime, keep a list of the best ethnic and health food restaurants in each city.

Since more and more research continues to surface about how much longer vegetarians live, it's definitely worth the effort to learn more about food and cooking. In the latest research, the additional years you gain as a vegetarian appear to be a minimum of six. That means you'll be eating at least an additional 6,570 meals.

(Y)our Future or
What's on the Horizon

A number of years ago, I read the definition of an American. It was someone who "would laugh at faith healers and spend hundreds of millions of dollars a year on fake reducing machines." That may be changing rapidly now, as *The New England Journal of Medicine* reported in a January 1993 article that one in three Americans turned to "unconventional therapy" and spent a whopping 10.7 billion dollars out-of-pocket for these visits.

The reasons for this upswing in interest are twofold. First of all, there is a growing dissatisfaction with current Western medical practices. Secondly, there is a greater concern and understanding of the real value of many traditional methods of healing. Whereas today's traditional doctor will ask where the pain is and give you something to take the pain away, the holistic doctor will ask you to identify physical, mental, and spiritual events taking place in your life that may be causing the pain. They look at the whole body. A very positive sign is that many of the tenets of holistic medicine practices are finding their way into Western medicine.

Herbal medicine is the oldest form of physical healing chronicled. More and more people are returning to this respected, ancient form of medicine. Indian and Chinese doctors have been using 4,000–5,000-year-old herbal prescriptions to strengthen the immune system. They must be effective or they would not continue using them.

The renaissance interest in herbal medicine

is a very positive one. Herbs are simply wild plants (medicinal vegetables). There are roughly 750,000 species of plants worldwide. Whereas drugs have a single effect and work on a single system, herbs have a wide range of responses. One herb may affect several organs at once. They are milder than drugs, which tend to overpower the body. Herbs speed healing and trigger the healing response (they activate white blood cells).

We seem to be making our future by going back to the past. Many disciplines of promoting good health are either resurfacing or gaining respectability—homeopathy, spiritual healing, hypnosis, acupuncture, yoga, meditation, fasting, etc. These alternative medicinal practices have helped people come to respect Grandma's remedies. Until the early 1900s and the increased population of medical doctors, most people healed themselves. Faith Popcorn, the futurist, commented that in the 21st century, "People will self-medicate and know how to choose the treatment that is right for them."

Our current generation has become obsessed with getting enough. The problem, however, is not that we don't get enough—it's one of excess. We overeat and overdrink. I would like to talk about one aspect of self-healing that is greatly misunderstood, and that is fasting.

13.1   Fasting

Fasting should be looked at as a physiological rest, not a deprivation. We give our head, legs, and eyes a rest, but seldom does our digestive system get a break. If it weren't for the fact that humans have to sleep, our stomach would be working nonstop.

The living body has one ability that is not possessed by any machine, and that is the ability to repair itself. When fasting, energy goes into healing instead of digesting. You get an accelerated waste removal. All of us have toxic buildup. Just as your home gets a special "spring cleaning" with extra time spent in doing a good, thorough job, so should our real homes (our bodies) get a good scrubbing. Fasting is a total regeneration and rejuvenation of all functions of the body. It is the oldest therapy known to humans that has been chronicled. Unfortunately, there is an irrational fear centered around fasting. At no time during a fast are we actually without food. In fact, most of us have plenty of reserves. The major fuel used is fat. Also, the body, in its wisdom, feeds off the least desirable tissue (the aged or diseased cells).

Most Westerners are so toxic that a water fast is much too stressful. Therefore, a juice fast is recommended. For first timers, experiment with a one-day fast and eventually work up to a five-day fast. For anything beyond five days, it is recommended that you have medical supervision. During fasting, you may feel cold and weak as you detoxify. It is important to get out and do some light exercise such as walking or swimming. Failure to exercise during a fast brings on fatigue. A note of caution: Children and pregnant women should never fast.

For the past ten years, I have tried to fast one day out of every ten. This may sound difficult, but in reality a lot of people come close to this anyway. The easiest fast is dinner to dinner. Since many people skip breakfast or lunch because they either slept in or are too busy, all that's needed is to skip one meal; the body will appreciate it.

I try to do the fast when traveling because our body is almost always quite vulnerable to getting sick at this time, due to the stress involved. This is an important time to keep your immune system high. Plan what would be the best time for you

271

to fast, so you can prepare mentally as well. And remember, you are not depriving your body of food, you are rewarding it with rest.

13.2   Recreation

Another important contribution to your health is recreation. We are so caught up in the pressures of our daily lives that we are robbing ourselves of the quality of our health and our life. We need to RE-CREATE, whether it's gardening, photography, tennis, hiking, boating, etc. Taking your cellular phone to the beach doesn't count. Recreation is so important that some countries have laws that force people to take true vacations. Try to incorporate at least fifteen minutes into your day for this essential aspect of good health.

What's Ahead

I'm often asked what's in store for us. I don't know, but I think it's safe to say that we're at least taking steps in the right direction toward healing both ourselves and our environment. At least we now understand more, and understanding is often the predecessor of doing.

Some trends are emerging, as sales of rice, legumes, fruits, and vegetables continue to rise significantly. There is a growing interest in organic farming. Even though the USDA has approximately 130 inspectors, only two deal with organic farming. Consumer interest and demand will change that. With organic farming, there will also be a greater focus on growing locally and eating locally to cut down on the energy and financial drain of long-distance transportation.

All of this would be aided greatly if the USDA would become more concerned with the health of the consumer than with the economic interests of the cattlemen and feed grain growers. Or, if they feel that the interests of the cattlemen are paramount, then the government should form a separate arm to oversee the welfare of the consumer. As it is now, the USDA has a major conflict of interest.

When Paul Obis began his publication of *Vegetarian Times* in November of 1974, he received only three orders. Today, it has over 480,000 subscribers—a very high number for a special interest publication. It won't be long before the circulation hits one million. As this vegetarian trend continues, it will be understood to be one of the most positive developments of our modern era.

An author and mother once wrote: "Writing a book is like the birth of a child. You are exhilarated when the child is born, but oh, was it painful." As I arrived at this last chapter, there was unquestionably great exhilaration. The pain was in caring so much that this book would make a difference. Since finishing school, I have become an avid reader. I can vividly remember those books that had a powerful impact on me, so, when writing this book, I truly wanted it to be a book that would be a "life-shaping experience" for its readers. Learning new truths forces us to shift and grow. They help us follow the conscience of our heart.

There are moments or events in everybody's life that provide opportunity to change old habits and behavior. I hope reading this book was one such moment for you. Whatever the case, I want to thank you for reading the book. I hope you'll share it with someone you love. And may I also thank my wife and daughters, who allowed me the quiet time to put it all together.

Appendices

VEGETARIAN COOKBOOKS
recommended by Peter and Lynn Burwash

Moosewood Cookbook
by Mollie Katzen
Ten Speed Press, 1992

The New Laurel's Kitchen
by Laurel Robertson
Ten Speed Press, 1996

The New Vegetarian Cookbook
by Gary Null
MacMillan Publishing Co., 1980

The McDougall Health-Supporting Cookbook
by Mary McDougall
New Win Publishing, 1986

Niki and David Golbeck's American Wholefoods Cuisine
by Nikki and David Goldbeck
New American Library Trade, 1995

The Compassionate Cook
by Ingrid E. Newkirk
Warner Books, 1993

Cooking With PETA: Great Vegan Recipes for a Compassionate Kitchen
by Ingrid E. Newkirk
PETA, 1997

Yamuna's Table: Healthful Vegetarian Cuisine Inspired by the Flavors of India
Yamuna Devi
Plume, 1995

Also, a wonderful monthly publication that is full of good vegetarian recipes is *Vegetarian Times*. You may write to them at Box 570, Oak Park, IL 60303. *Veggie Life*, from the Vegetarian Resource Group, is another. PO Box 1463 Baltimore MD 21203.

There are hundreds of vegetarian cookbooks available today, and these are just a few to get you started. You can find them in most health food stores and book stores.

RESOURCES

r A New America
n Robbins
int Publishing, 1987

ning Our Health
n Robbins
amer, 1996

s Vegetarians And Their Favorite Recipes: Lives And Lore
Buddha To The Beatles
an Berry
orean Books, 1993

an Ornish's Program For Reversing Heart Disease
an Ornish
om House, 1990

y of Stress
er G. Hanson
ws and McMeel, 1987

d Beef: The Rise and Fall of the Cattle Culture
emy Rifkin
e, 1993

279

Eat Right - Live Longer: Using The Power of Foods To Age Proof Your Body
by Neal Barnard
Harmony Books, 1995

Mind, Body, And Sport: the Mind-Body Guide To Lifelong Fitness And Your Personal Best
by John Douillard
Crown Publishing, 1995

Garden Cuisine, Heal Yourself And The Planet Through Lowfat, Meatless Eating
by Paul F. Wenner
Simon & Schuster, 1997

Superpigs and Wondercorn: The Brave New World of Biotechnology and Where It May All Lead
by Michael W. Fox
Lyons and Burford, 1992

The Boundless Circle: Caring For Creatures And Creation
by Michael W. Fox
Quest Books, 1996

Eating With Conscience: The Bioethics of Food
by Michael W. Fox
New Sage Press, 1997

The Vegetarian Revolution: A Commentary And Cookbook
by Giorgio Cerquetti
Torchlight Publishing, 1997

Diet For Transcendence: Vegetarianism And The World Religions
by Steven Rosen
Torchlight Publishing, 1997

ORGANIZATIONS

San Francisco Vegetarian Society
PO Box 27153 San Francisco CA 94127

Vegetarian Resource Group
PO Box 1463 Baltimore MD 21203

Vegetarian Resource Center
PO Box 38-1068 Cambridge MA 02238-1068

EarthSave
706 Frederick St Santa Cruz CA 95062

Vegetarian Society Inc.
PO Box 34427 Los Angeles CA 90034

FARM
Box 30654 Bethesda MD 20824

Vegetarians International
PO Box 45 Badger CA 93603

International Society for Cow Protection (ISCOWP)
RD 1 NBU #28 Moundsville WV 26041

The Humane Society of the United States
2100 L St NW Washington DC 20037

People for the Ethical Treatment of Animals (PETA)
501 Front St Norfolk VA 23510

North American Vegetarian Association
PO Box 72 Dolgeville, NY 13329

About The Author

Peter Burwash first became prominent in the 1970s as a young professional on the international tennis circuit and soon became well known for his fierce determination, all-out performance, and passion for the game.

Peter is now recognized as one of the top tennis coaches in the world, having coached in 134 countries on five continents. Peter won nineteen international singles and doubles titles and became a Canadian champion and Davis Cup player during his years playing the international circuit. He shares his tennis knowledge with a nationwide audience on CBS radio, as an instruction editor for *Tennis* magazine, and as a television commentator and analyst. *Tennis Industry* magazine recognized Peter as "one of the most influential tennis teachers of the past two decades."

As a best selling-author, his book *Tennis for Life* was translated into several languages, revolutionizing the game of tennis around the world. A second book, *Total Tennis,* soon followed, as did award-winning instructional videos, which many consider a "must buy" for any tennis library.

His fifth book, *The Key to Great Leadership— Rediscovering the Principles of Outstanding Service,* was endorsed by leadership giant Steven Covey and Brian Tracy, author and motivational speaker. It is a compilation of Peter's research and life experiences, explaining why everyone should consider himself/herself a leader.

In 1975, Peter founded Peter Burwash International (PBI), the world's largest and most successful international tennis management firm. Listing PBI as "one of the ten best-managed companies in America," Dr. James O'Toole, in his book *Vanguard Management,* stated that PBI "may well be a forerunner of a class of entirely new service organizations."

Traveling over ten million miles in the last twenty-five years has not slowed the man who previously recorded the highest fitness index of any Canadian athlete. Peter Burwash is also a certified nutritionist and uniquely qualified to present this book, his sixth: *Total Health: The Next Level.*

Peter is sought after internationally as a speaker and gives over one hundred speeches and seminars each year on a variety of topics, ranging from health and fitness to service and leadership.

For more information on Peter Burwash's availability as a speaker, contact Torchlight Publishing.

PETER BURWASH

LIFE ENRICHMENT LIBRARY

If you liked this book by Peter Burwash you
may be interested in the others in his Life
Enrichment Library. Please take a look at
Peter's four other titles on the following
pages and use the ordering information at
the back of the book to purchase further
copies.

Special prices are available for bulk orders.

How You Can Become a Great Leader

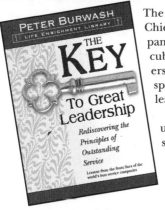

PETER BURWASH
LIFE ENRICHMENT LIBRARY
THE
KEY
To Great
Leadership
Rediscovering the
Principles of
Outstanding
Service
Lessons from the front lines of the
world's best service companies

The President of the United States, the Chief Executive of a Fortune 500 company, and the mother of an eight year old cub scout are each in a position of leadership. But how do you develop those special qualities that bring success as a leader?

The Key shows clearly and simply the underlying principles that make for successful leadership.

Whether you're Chairman of the Board or a mother of three, in *The Key* you will find a wealth of information to enrich your life.

"Inspirational and compelling bite-size quotes illustrated by motivational stories in two key competitive advantages of the future—service and leadership."
– Dr. Steven Covey, chairman of Covey Leadership Center and author of *The Seven Habits of Highly Effective People.*

"Peter's firm is the biggest and best of its kind in the world because he follows the precepts outlined in *The Key*. He knows how to create a high-trust culture and a high-energy work force and he tells you concisely and clearly, from experience, how it's done."
– from the foreword by Isadore Sharp, founder and chairman of Four Seasons hotels and resorts.

Paperback 4.75 x 6.5 inches, 240 pages, $9.95
ISBN 10: 0-9779785-0-8
ISBN 13: 978-09779785-0-5
See back page for ordering information

Dear Teenager

NAVIGATING THE TURBULANT YEARS AND BUILDING A FOUNDATION FOR A MEANINGFUL LIFE

By Peter Burwash

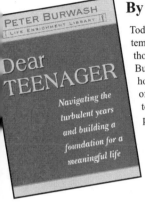

Today's teenagers face an alarming array of hurdles, temptations, and confusing signals. After spending thousands of hours listening to teenagers, Peter Burwash, in a straightforward yet sympathetic style hones in on their major problems and concerns and offers the knowledge of his own life experiences to help teens through this difficult transitional period. Helpful to parents and mentors of teenagers as well, *Dear Teenager* is a guide to growing up healthy and whole physically, mentally, and spiritually.

A few of Peter Burwash's surefire tips for teens:

"When you get up in the morning, you really only have one major decision to make, and that is whether you are going to have a good attitude or a bad attitude."

"We tend to become the type of person with whom we associate. Do your utmost to choose your friends wisely."

"Most adults look back on their teenage years and say, 'I wish I had known then what I know now' why? Because knowledge eliminates fear. And during our years as teenagers, there's so much anxiety and fear that some extra knowledge could go a long way to help paddle through the waves of insecurity."

"Adversity and struggle are such wonderful teachers. Adversity often introduces us To ourselves, and struggle makes us appreciate the end result so much more."

Paperback 4.75 x 6.5 inches, 240 pages, $9.95
ISBN 10: 0-9779785-2-4 ISBN 13: 978-09779785-2-6
See back page for ordering information

Take charge of your life!

**"A blend of practical wisdom
and a depth of experience to
teach us how to take charge
of every aspect of our lives."**
—from the foreword by
Lee Iacocca

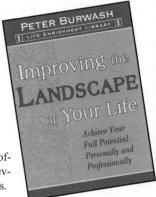

Improving the Landscape of Your Life offers a fresh, practical approach to achieving new levels of personal effectiveness.

Peter Burwash reveals twelve essential
habits for succeeding and understanding true happiness.

The happiest people are those who try to help others and who don't
necessarily have the best of everything, but they make the best of
everything they have.

Although Peter's book is presented in bite size chapters, don't let this
fool you. Inside you'll find twelve very powerful and practical lessons on how to take charge of every aspect of your life.

Paperback 4.75 x 6.5 inches, 128 pages, $9.95
ISBN 10: 0-9779785-1-6 ; ISBN 13: 978-09779785-1-9
See back page for ordering information

Becoming the Master of Your D-A-S-H

You and I don't play much of a role in our entrance into this life and we have minimal say about how and when we'll depart. Yet we have a major influence on the time and experiences in between, written as the dash (—) between the dates of our births and deaths.

With personal anecdotes, real-izations, and sage advice from enlightened people, past and present (who have done well at mastering their D-A-S-Hes), Peter Burwash offers us a dozen fundamental guidelines for improving our precious journey.

Here are just a few samples:

- Develop an attitude of gratitude.
- Slow down and stop running "everyday-a-thons".
- Life never goes in a straight line, nor should it.
- Being the richest person in the cemetery isn't so important.
- An ego trip is a journey nowhere.
- The best things in life aren't things.

Whether you find Peter's advice an alarming wake up call or the encouraging words of a kind and experienced well-wisher, one thing is for sure—this is one of the most cogent 'How To' books you'll find for making the most of this mysterious blessing we call life.

Paperback 4.75 x 6.5 inches,144 pages, $9.95
ISBN 10: 0-9779785-4-0 ISBN 13: 978-0-9779785-4-0
See back page for ordering information

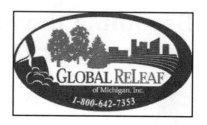

Torchlight Publishing recognizes that maintaining a sustainable ecosystem is vital to our planet's future. We support the replanting of trees by donating money to the Global Releaf campaign of American Forests for the replanting of two trees for every tree we use in the production of our books and other materials. American Forests has planted tens of millions of trees in hundreds of ecosystem restoration projects throughout the United States and around the world.

We encourage our readers to support this important program. You can make a tangible difference that will help to improve the environment for generations to come. For more information, please visit their website at: www.globalreleaf.com

ORDER FORM

CALL & ORDER NOW!

Telephone orders: Call 1-888-TORCHLT (1-888-867-2458)

Have your VISA or MasterCard ready

Fax orders: (559)-337-2354

Postal orders: PO Box 52, Badger CA 93603

Web orders: www.torchlight.com

Please send the following. I understand I may return any
books for a full refund—for any reason, no questions asked.

❑   *The Key to Great Leadership* $9.95.................... No. of copies _____

❑   *Total Health* $9.95... No. of copies _____

❑   *Dear Teenager* $9.95... No. of copies _____

❑   *Improving the Landscape of Your Life* $9.95...... No. of copies _____

❑   *Becoming the Master of Your Dash* $9.95........... No. of copies _____

Please add my name to your mailing list so I may receive information on
future books published by Torchlight.

Company _____

Name _____

City _____ State_____ Zip _____

Country _____Phone _____

Sales tax: California residents add 8.25%
Shipping and handling: Book rate: USA and Canada $2.00 for first book and $1.50
for each additional book. Foreign countries $2.50 for first book, $2.00 for each additional book. (Surface shipping may take 6-8 weeks. Foreign orders please allow 6-8
weeks for delivery) Priority Air Mail (USA only) $3.50 per book.

Payment: ❑   Check/money order enclosed   ❑   Credit card

❑   VISA   ❑   Master Card

Card #_____ Exp.date _____

Name on card_____

Signature _____